Menopause in Perspective

Phi. a Pigache has been a journalist and writer for more than 30 years, star on local newspapers and women's magazines, moving to national news pers, radio and television and, more recently, becoming a freelance medic science writer. She has worked on the *Sunday Times, Daily Mail, Daily l rror* and *The Guardian*, and for ITN and BBC science features.

Sh tarted to write about medicine chiefly because she was married to a doc . (Her own educational background is in modern languages and the th atre.) She has contributed to consumer health pages and journals hea th professionals for 20 years and has won awards for her medical nalism and also for her fiction. She is currently the honorary secretary f Medical Journalists' Association and editor of their journal, the *MJA* vs.

o has written consumer health books on lupus, arthritis, Attention Ne Hyperactivity Disorder (ADHD) and how to be a healthy weight.

Sl ook for Sheldon Press, *Living with Rheumatoid Arthritis*, was com-Defic in the 2005 MJA Open Consumer Book Awards. She has one Her l, two children, three grandchildren and two cats. She lives in mer nd paints and gardens in her spare time.

hu'

Su

Overcoming Common Problems Series

Selected titles

A full list of titles is available from Sheldon Press,
36 Causton Street, London SW1P 4ST and on our website at
www.sheldonpress.co.uk

The Assertiveness Handbook
Mary Hartley

Assertiveness: Step by step
Dr Windy Dryden and Daniel Constantinou

Backache: What you need to know
Dr David Delvin

Body Language: What you need to know
David Cohen

The Cancer Survivor's Handbook
Dr Terry Priestman

The Candida Diet Book
Karen Brody

The Chronic Fatigue Healing Diet
Christine Craggs-Hinton

The Chronic Pain Diet Book
Neville Shone

Cider Vinegar
Margaret Hills

The Complete Carer's Guide
Bridget McCall

The Confidence Book
Gordon Lamont

Confidence Works
Gladeana McMahon

Coping Successfully with Pain
Neville Shone

Coping Successfully with Panic Attacks
Shirley Trickett

Coping Successfully with Period Problems
Mary-Claire Mason

Coping Successfully with Psoriasis
Christine Craggs-Hinton

Coping Successfully with Ulcerative Colitis
Peter Cartwright

Coping Successfully with Varicose Veins
Christine Craggs-Hinton

Coping Successfully with Your Hiatus Hernia
Dr Tom Smith

Coping Successfully with Your Irritable Bowel
Rosemary Nicol

Coping When Your Child Has Cerebral Palsy
Jill Eckersley

Coping with Age-related Memory Loss
Dr Tom Smith

Coping with Birth Trauma and Postnatal Depression
Lucy Jolin

Coping with Bowel Cancer
Dr Tom Smith

Coping with Candida
Shirley Trickett

Coping with Chemotherapy
Dr Terry Priestman

Coping with Chronic Fatigue
Trudie Chalder

Coping with Coeliac Disease
Karen Brody

Coping with Compulsive Eating
Ruth Searle

Coping with Diabetes in Childhood and Adolescence
Dr Philippa Kaye

Coping with Diverticulitis
Peter Cartwright

Coping with Down's Syndrome
Fiona Marshall

Coping with Dyspraxia
Jill Eckersley

Coping with Eating Disorders and Body Image
Christine Craggs-Hinton

Coping with Epilepsy in Children and Young People
Susan Elliot-Wright

Coping with Family Stress
Dr Peter Cheevers

Coping with Gout
Christine Craggs-Hinton

Coping with Hay Fever
Christine Craggs-Hinton

Coping with Headaches and Migraine
Alison Frith

Overcoming Common Problems Series

Coping with Hearing Loss
Christine Craggs-Hinton

Coping with Heartburn and Reflux
Dr Tom Smith

Coping with Kidney Disease
Dr Tom Smith

Coping with Life after Stroke
Dr Mareeni Raymond

Coping with Macular Degeneration
Dr Patricia Gilbert

Coping with a Mid-life Crisis
Derek Milne

Coping with PMS
Dr Farah Ahmed and Dr Emma Cordle

Coping with Polycystic Ovary Syndrome
Christine Craggs-Hinton

Coping with Postnatal Depression
Sandra L. Wheatley

Coping with Radiotherapy
Dr Terry Priestman

Coping with a Stressed Nervous System
Dr Kenneth Hambly and Alice Muir

Coping with Suicide
Maggie Helen

Coping with Tinnitus
Christine Craggs-Hinton

Coping with Type 2 Diabetes
Susan Elliot-Wright

Coping with Your Partner's Death: Your bereavement guide
Geoff Billings

The Depression Diet Book
Theresa Cheung

Depression: Healing emotional distress
Linda Hurcombe

Depressive Illness
Dr Tim Cantopher

Eating for a Healthy Heart
Robert Povey, Jacqui Morrell and Rachel Povey

Every Woman's Guide to Digestive Health
Jill Eckersley

The Fertility Handbook
Dr Philippa Kaye

The Fibromyalgia Healing Diet
Christine Craggs-Hinton

Free Your Life from Fear
Jenny Hare

Free Yourself from Depression
Colin and Margaret Sutherland

A Guide to Anger Management
Mary Hartley

Heal the Hurt: How to forgive and move on
Dr Ann Macaskill

Helping Children Cope with Anxiety
Jill Eckersley

Helping Children Cope with Grief
Rosemary Wells

How to Approach Death
Julia Tugendhat

How to be a Healthy Weight
Philippa Pigache

How to Beat Pain
Christine Craggs-Hinton

How to Cope with Difficult People
Alan Houel and Christian Godefroy

How to Get the Best from Your Doctor
Dr Tom Smith

How to Manage Chronic Fatigue
Christine Craggs-Hinton

How to Stop Worrying
Dr Frank Tallis

How to Talk to Your Child
Penny Oates

Hysterectomy: Is it right for you?
Janet Wright

The IBS Healing Plan
Theresa Cheung

Letting Go of Anxiety and Depression
Dr Windy Dryden

Living with Angina
Dr Tom Smith

Living with Asperger Syndrome
Dr Joan Gomez

Living with Autism
Fiona Marshall

Living with Bipolar Disorder
Dr Neel Burton

Living with Birthmarks and Blemishes
Gordon Lamont

Living with Crohn's Disease
Dr Joan Gomez

Living with Eczema
Jill Eckersley

Living with Fibromyalgia
Christine Craggs-Hinton

Living with Food Intolerance
Alex Gazzola

Overcoming Common Problems Series

Living with Gluten Intolerance
Jane Feinmann

Living with Grief
Dr Tony Lake

Living with Loss and Grief
Julia Tugendhat

Living with Osteoarthritis
Dr Patricia Gilbert

Living with Osteoporosis
Dr Joan Gomez

Living with Physical Disability and Amputation
Dr Keren Fisher

Living with Rheumatoid Arthritis
Philippa Pigache

Living with Schizophrenia
Dr Neel Burton and Dr Phil Davison

Living with a Seriously Ill Child
Dr Jan Aldridge

Living with Sjögren's Syndrome
Sue Dyson

Living with Type 1 Diabetes
Dr Tom Smith

Losing a Child
Linda Hurcombe

The Multiple Sclerosis Diet Book
Tessa Buckley

Osteoporosis: Prevent and treat
Dr Tom Smith

Overcome Your Fear of Flying
Professor Robert Bor, Dr Carina Eriksen and
Margaret Oakes

Overcoming Agoraphobia
Melissa Murphy

Overcoming Anorexia
Professor J. Hubert Lacey, Christine Craggs-Hinton
and Kate Robinson

Overcoming Anxiety
Dr Windy Dryden

Overcoming Back Pain
Dr Tom Smith

Overcoming Depression
Dr Windy Dryden and Sarah Opie

Overcoming Emotional Abuse
Susan Elliot-Wright

Overcoming Hurt
Dr Windy Dryden

Overcoming Insomnia
Susan Elliot-Wright

Overcoming Jealousy
Dr Windy Dryden

**Overcoming Panic and Related Anxiety
Disorders**
Margaret Hawkins

Overcoming Procrastination
Dr Windy Dryden

Overcoming Shyness and Social Anxiety
Ruth Searle

Overcoming Tiredness and Exhaustion
Fiona Marshall

Reducing Your Risk of Cancer
Dr Terry Priestman

Safe Dieting for Teens
Linda Ojeda

**Self-discipline: How to get it and how to
keep it**
Dr Windy Dryden

The Self-Esteem Journal
Alison Waines

Simplify Your Life
Naomi Saunders

Sinusitis: Steps to healing
Dr Paul Carson

Stammering: Advice for all ages
Renée Byrne and Louise Wright

Stress-related Illness
Dr Tim Cantopher

Ten Steps to Positive Living
Dr Windy Dryden

Think Your Way to Happiness
Dr Windy Dryden and Jack Gordon

The Thinking Person's Guide to Happiness
Ruth Searle

**Tranquillizers and Antidepressants: When to
take them, how to stop**
Professor Malcolm Lader

The Traveller's Good Health Guide
Dr Ted Lankester

Treating Arthritis Diet Book
Margaret Hills

Treating Arthritis: The drug-free way
Margaret Hills and Christine Horner

**Treating Arthritis: More ways to a drug-free
life**
Margaret Hills

Understanding Obsessions and Compulsions
Dr Frank Tallis

When Someone You Love Has Dementia
Susan Elliot-Wright

When Someone You Love Has Depression
Barbara Baker

Overcoming Common Problems

Menopause in Perspective

PHILIPPA PIGACHE

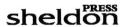

First published in Great Britain in 2010

Sheldon Press
36 Causton Street
London SW1P 4ST

The author and publisher have made every effort to ensure that the
external website and email addresses included in this book are correct and
up to date at the time of going to press. The author and publisher are not
responsible for the content, quality or continuing accessibility of the sites.

British Library Cataloguing-in-Publication Data
A catalogue record for this book is available from the British Library

ISBN 978-1-84709-055-3

1 3 5 7 9 10 8 6 4 2

Typeset by Fakenham Photosetting Ltd, Fakenham, Norfolk
Printed in Great Britain by Ashford Colour Press

Produced on paper from sustainable forests

Contents

Introduction		ix
1	What's happening to me?	1
2	Natural event or historic accident?	11
3	When menopause?	20
4	Do we, don't we, treat the menopause?	27
5	Making a personal choice: is HRT for you?	39
6	The menopause and your heart	49
7	The menopause and cancer	59
8	The menopause and your bones	68
9	Meanwhile, in another part of the body	77
10	Managing the rest of your life	86
Epilogue		97
Glossary		99
Appendix		106
Further reading		108
Useful addresses and websites		109
Index		111

For my mother, who came through and had a full postmenopause life despite everything

Introduction

You have picked up this book almost certainly either because you are going through the menopause or because you see it on the horizon. I am writing it from the calm uplands beyond. From where I stand I see the menopause as a relatively brief interval – a pause – marking a change. (It is often called the Change of Life.) To be more precise, it is not so much a change of life as a change of fertility. Some women approach the menopause with dread, seeing it as The End of Life as We Know it. But it's not. Let me offer you to start with three useful thoughts that have informed me in writing this book, and that may also help you, I hope, in going through the menopause.

- The menopause is not an illness.
- All women, provided they don't die young, go through it (another reason for insisting that it is not regarded as an illness), and survive.
- And finally, be an optimist: more than half your adult life is yet to come.

When you compare life before and after the menopause – that is, ever since you started periods (the *menarche* as it is called), not before that – the most dramatic difference is that the latter period is inevitably a great deal less eventful. Youth and middle age can be turbulent times. By the time you reach the menopause most of the major turning points in life are behind you. You've done childbirth, marriage (or not, as the case may be), setting up house, career. If you've developed the latter, unless you are into politics you are probably at the peak of your powers. Whatever you have done with your life up to now, you almost certainly know yourself and what you expect from life pretty well. This should help you go through the menopause with the minimum of inconvenience, and emerge the other side positive and optimistic about the rest of your life. The average British woman has 30 years ahead of her after the menopause: make the most of it.

It wasn't until the nineteenth century that most women lived long enough to reach the menopause. Serious study of the condition probably dates from about 80 years ago – within living memory. And in that time attitudes to as well as treatments for the menopause have changed radically. We are more open about all aspects of human reproduction and sexuality these days. We don't treat 'women's problems' as something slightly embarrassing – or worse, shameful – and just sweep them under the carpet. My mother went through the menopause with no mention of it. I didn't even know the meaning of the word until I started to write about health a few years later. Medicines and attitudes to them have also changed. We now have drugs for things often referred to as 'lifestyle choices' as well as illness; most notably contraception, which uses some of the same manufactured hormones prescribed to treat the symptoms of the menopause. There are still people who think it sissy to take aspirin, who regard anything as unnatural as artificial hormones as anathema and who are persuaded that since the menopause is natural it must be endured. There are also those who adopt a 'plague on all your drugs' attitude and turn instead to what are known as alternative or complementary treatments. It's an understandable response to the way that new drugs are often greeted as the greatest thing since sliced bread only later to be revealed as somewhat less revolutionary, or dogged with unwelcome side effects.

This is what has happened to *hormone replacement therapy* (HRT) – the drugs prescribed to treat the symptoms of the menopause. When it was first discovered how much relief the combination of artificial hormones could provide for the short-term but often devastating symptoms some women suffered – the dreaded hot flushes that could reduce her to a hot wet flannel in front of a class of 30 children or in the middle of an important board meeting – and in addition that it could protect them from that old woman's scourge brittle bones, women couldn't believe their luck. They rushed from the doctor's surgery to the chemist clutching their prescriptions and within days were feeling better. So much better that many were tempted to believe that those artificial hormones contained the secret of eternal youth: unwrinkled skin, thick hair, strong bones and an enthusiasm for sex, in addition to freedom from hot flushes.

But after that initial reaction the bad stories began to come in. A whole raft of research studies that looked at HRT long term – the work at Wake Forest University, the Nurses Study, and most particularly the more thorough Women's Health Initiative (WHI) in the USA and the Million Women study in the UK (you will become familiar with the acronyms that identify them during the course of this book) – began to appear and newspapers, magazines and television carried scary stories linking these drugs to heart attack, stroke, breast cancer and other health hazards. What made it worse was that the studies didn't all sing from the same hymn sheet. Some studies actually seemed to contradict each other and even the medical profession became divided. You might get one view from your GP and quite another from the specialist at the hospital, or the practice nurse in the clinic. Never mind mood swings or hot flushes, the stories themselves were enough to make you feel quite giddy.

Even today it is very difficult to find really balanced advice on HRT. The medical profession remains divided, with gynaecologists tending to be more pro than endocrinologists, according to Tom Parkhill in the journal *Endocrinology* in 2006. He writes that on the internet he found a chorus of horror stories, a mushroom-growth of so-called alternative treatments, but no consistent messages from authoritative bodies such as the Medicines and Healthcare Regulatory Agency (MHRA), the medical Royal Colleges or the British Menopause Society (whose 2006 book, *The Menopause: What you need to know*, referenced at the back of this book, gives factual and rather scary health data but doesn't really help you decide what you personally should do). The Amarant Trust, the main patient group for HRT in the UK, has a useful website (listed at the back of this book) but their telephone helpline was suspended in 2005 due to lack of funds.

Good advice is hard to find, and if you read on you will begin to see why. There is no one-size-fits-all for coping with the menopause. It is the aim of this book to help you see through the temporary symptoms of the menopause and make the most of the rest of your life. I hope to sort the science from the hype; to examine the health risks and benefits revealed by the controversial studies of recent years (which are still being interpreted), so that you can make decisions about what treatment is appropriate for you. One thing the studies reveal is what, deep down, we all know anyway.

Not all women are the same: some inevitably are more at risk in the menopause and postmenopause than others. Knowing where you fall in this risk spectrum is essential to making wise choices as to treatment and life-behaviour. The other thing revealed is about the timing and the dosage that is effective with HRT. In a nutshell, it should be started early and tapered off as soon as reasonably comfortable and practical.

How to read this book

You can, if you wish, read this book from beginning to end. Or you can use it to zero in on what concerns you about the menopause: the symptoms, risks, or long-term health aspects. The first chapter provides a glimpse into the menopause as a personal but variable experience; one of the case histories may be close to your own. It goes on to provide a brief introduction to how the hormones that govern fertility work in the body and the changes that take place during the menopause – the basic physiology. You can skip this if the science is less important to you than the practicalities, but it will help you understand why hormones are so important to your health and well-being. In Chapter 2 I try to put the menopause into a wider perspective – in history and in different cultures. This is not just an academic activity because the way a condition is regarded socially affects the way it is experienced. It also helps you, as an individual, to adopt constructive attitudes to what is happening to you. Chapter 3 discusses the timing of the menopause, which is not as straightforward as you may think, and Chapter 4 reviews the treatments available for menopausal symptoms, including the many different forms of HRT, and the alternatives. Chapter 5 goes into more details about studies of HRT in an attempt to help you decide whether it is right for you, for your individual symptoms and your individual health profile. Then follow four chapters that look at the way various health risks in later life – heart disease, cancer, deteriorating bones and skin – are affected by the loss of oestrogen that occurs at the menopause; who is most at risk of what, and how HRT affects these conditions. They make rather grim reading and depending on your personal risk profile, you may choose to skip those that don't concern you. Finally, Chapter 10 focuses upon the long-term view – a perspective – not just of treatments you may choose to traverse the menopause but the attitudes and behaviours you can adopt that will help you through this time of turbulence and on to the calm uplands beyond.

Difficult words are explained in the text and those printed in *italic* when first they appear (though not throughout the text) are also listed in the Glossary at the end of the book, where you will also find useful addresses, websites and further reading. Some interesting information not essential to understanding the themes of the book is picked out in separate boxes.

1

What's happening to me?

My mother stood in the kitchen holding a mop and wept. Mandy, our golden retriever, had given birth to eight pups. They were so fat their legs could barely touch the floor and they were not house-trained. They skidded all over the kitchen floor piddling on sheets of pee-soaked newspaper. The rest of the family thought it hilarious. It reduced my mum to tears. It was only years later, when I started to write about health, that I realized that she must have been going through the menopause. We thought it was the stress of the puppies – paddling through their feeding bowls and peeing all over the place. Her generation thought that their children should not even know how old they were, let alone discuss personal things like periods, or periods that stop.

Bursting into tears at the drop of a fat puppy may not be one of the classic symptoms of the menopause, but mood swings, being irritable and becoming depressed are. That winter she would also occasionally throw off all her clothes and step under the shower. With hindsight she must have been having hot flushes.

I realized that my friend Maria had hit the menopause ahead of me when I begged a Tampax off her in an emergency and she told me she hadn't used them for nearly a year. By this time I was more focused. 'But aren't you having horrible hot flushes? Do you still feel like having sex? Have you started to put on weight?' I asked with concern. 'You know, I really haven't noticed,' she replied casually. 'They just sort of tailed off; became shorter and less frequent until I realized they had stopped.'

My generation, unlike my mother's, shares details of their health and personal experience with friends. My daughter's generation now puts its symptoms on the internet on Facebook.

Caroline writes: 'My periods were going haywire – more frequent and lasting longer, and I was feeling so tired but I never thought it could be the menopause, after all, I was only 42. My youngest child was only four years old! Anyway, after six months of getting more irritable and weepy for no reason I started getting hot flushes in the daytime so I went to my doctor. She was very understanding and recommended HRT. I'm quite good at taking tablets so I tried those first. It took a couple of months to get used to HRT; at first my breasts were very tender – a bit like early pregnancy – but my doctor had warned me that could happen and it's all settled down now. I feel much more like my old self; and at least I know when my periods will happen and they don't drag on for days.'

Jennifer was alerted to the risks of the menopause by the history of her mother. 'I decided to start HRT when I reached the menopause because my mother has bad osteoporosis and broke her hip last year. I've done quite a bit of reading and know that osteoporosis can be prevented now. And I certainly don't want to have the back pain and hip problems my mother has suffered. So as soon as my periods stopped a year ago I asked my doctor for advice. It was a decision we made together. We decided to go for patches because they're so easy and suit my lifestyle. My periods aren't bad at all but as soon as I am old enough – around age 54 my doctor says – I will change to a no-bleed type of HRT, as I don't really want to go on having a regular bleed if I can avoid it with different medication. I didn't really have any menopausal symptoms but I know this is doing my bones good and will prevent the awful problems my mother has.'

These two women were recommended to take HRT, but the next patient received quite different advice, although she had similar symptoms. 'Age 55; symptoms: ten months since her last period, feeling disorientation, vexation, agitation and irascibility. Overwhelmed with melancholy and unease in the chest; suffering from hot flushes, insomnia and often alarmed by nightmares; difficult *defecation*.' She had come to a Chinese medicine specialist and was prescribed a concoction of 14 roots, seeds and other active herbal remedies. If a condition is not fatal – and we must be grateful for the fact that the menopause is at most uncomfortable – the treatment that may be offered, or sought, is more varied.

More symptoms and unpleasant coincidences

Browse the internet and you will find even more symptoms of the menopause. Jane's periods became heavy and irregular. One had been so severe that she had been confined to the house for several days within reach of the bathroom, waking two or three times a night to change her towel. When she went to her doctor she discovered that she had become *anaemic* – that's when you don't have enough red blood cells to carry the oxygen around your body adequately. It happens when you lose a lot of blood. The GP prescribed tablets to boost her red blood cells and HRT to regulate her periods. Joanna's periods were still regular but she had become extremely moody and begun to get the most frightful *premenstrual tension*. In addition, sexual intercourse had started to become uncomfortable for her because her vagina was so dry, and this was causing problems with her husband.

Sometimes a woman may come to her GP about symptoms that do not at first appear to be directly related to the menopause. She comes because she is putting on weight; because she is depressed; because she can't sleep; or because of the sort of family problem that often crops up for women around the age of 50 – her teenage kids are going off the rails; her husband has had an affair; she's lost her job and feels that she is too old to get another one; her ageing mother can't look after herself and might have to go into a home or even come and live with them. The menopause often coincides with a host of other problems.

Short-term and long-term symptoms

Strictly speaking, there is a precise medical definition of when the menopause takes place. It is when a woman has not had a period for 12 months. The average age at which women cross this finishing line these days is 52. And for women like my friend Maria, that is almost all it is. Sanitary towels are no longer on your shopping list. But for most women the menopause stretches over several years, and in terms of symptoms experienced, it starts before and it continues beyond the event itself. Some changes, like loss of bone density or thinning skin, are there for the rest of your life.

First come the short-term ones that surround the event itself: heavy periods, hot flushes, moods, drying up of secretions in the vagina, and ultimately, of course, the end of periods. Many of these are unpleasant and disruptive, but none is fatal. Later come the long-term symptoms following the physical changes heralded by the menopause: changes caused principally by the body producing less of the *hormones* that govern the monthly cycle. These changes are permanent, and some can be serious. They affect bones, joints, blood vessels and more. Doctors take them seriously and so should you. Again, they don't affect all women after the menopause; but they do affect more women in that age group.

And here, of course, we come back to something else that muddies the waters around the menopause. It is almost impossible to separate this event from things that happen *as* you get older, or *because* you get older – children leaving home, aches and pains, developing wrinkles and feeling too tired for sex. But we will try.

Why is all this happening to me?

The symptoms of the menopause are the result of the physical changes going on in your body at this time. You don't have to understand all the medical science, but it does help you understand and manage the troublesome symptoms if you know something of the physical causes of the symptoms. Let's start with the litany of disturbed mood. Quoted above we have tears, irritability, tension, disorientation, vexation, agitation, irascibility and melancholy. It's probably no surprise to learn that it all comes back to hormones.

Hormones – and there are a great many – are chemical messengers in the body. They control a vast range of different processes, physical and emotional. They work in conjunction with one another, in sequence, stimulating each other, and counteracting each other. A little less of one or too much of another and the delicate balance of processes going on in your body goes haywire. This is what happens at the menopause to the hormones that are in charge of your monthly fertility cycle. And this is why your emotions may also be in turmoil.

The family of oestrogens

There are several different sorts of oestrogens at work in the body, which perform slightly different functions.

- *Oestradiol* is the most powerful form of oestrogen. Produced in the ovaries, it sets off the physical changes that herald fertility at puberty and it drops right off when a woman is no longer fertile at the end of the menopause. Production rises in the first half of the menstrual cycle and results in the bulking up of the womb lining – the *endometrium* – in preparation for a fertilized egg. A small amount of oestradiol is produced by fat cells elsewhere in the body and in men. (This is important when discussing cancer risk after the menopause.)
- *Oestrone* is a weaker form of oestrogen but it is the main form found in your body after the menopause. Oestradiol can be converted into oestrone (they are in the same family).
- *Oestriol* (pay attention now, all three words are terribly alike) is the form of oestrogen only produced in any quantity during pregnancy. At that time the levels found in the mother's blood are important indicators of the developing baby's health, but it is not significant when discussing the menopause.

The three forms of oestrogen above are all naturally occurring (made by your own body). You will come across one other kind of oestrogen: the synthetic kinds used to treat a deficiency of the natural kind in women unable to produce their own, or at the menopause to alleviate some of the unpleasant symptoms. They are sometimes referred to as conjugated oestrogens. Conjugated means joined, and implies that they are assembled in the laboratory rather than in the body.

The most significant hormone for those encountering the menopause is *oestrogen* – or oestrogens, in the plural, because there are several different sorts of oestrogen. (See box, *The family of oestrogens*.) Oestrogen is the ringmaster where fertility is concerned: it both sets the ball rolling at puberty and calls a halt at the menopause. Some might say that oestrogen is the most quintessentially female of hormones, although it is not exclusive to women; men produce it too but in smaller quantities.

But the role of oestrogen extends way beyond fertility. It affects emotions, heat regulation, blood pressure, the levels of various fats in the blood, bone density, brain function and cancer risk. It is an exceedingly important hormone, and one of its principal functions is to stimulate the growth and multiplication of cells. It is the production of oestrogen in a teenage girl's body that causes her breasts and body hair to develop, the lining of her vagina to become stronger and more resilient, and her womb, ovaries and the *Fallopian tubes* (which carry unfertilized eggs, *ova*, singular *ovum*, to the womb) to mature in preparation for the release of eggs (*ovulation*). Once this maturation is complete, monthly periods start and this regular process will continue, controlled by the rise and fall of several different hormones, throughout her fertile life unless pregnancy or contraceptive pills interrupt it.

Other players in the menstrual cycle

Another key hormone in the menstrual cycle is *progesterone*. Its principal job is to prepare the body for pregnancy. Two more hormones play a role in the reproductive cycle because they kick-start oestrogen production, and it is worth explaining them even though they are less important when talking about the menopause. These are *follicle-stimulating hormone* (FSH) and *luteinizing hormone* (LH), both of which are made in the *pituitary gland* – a tiny gland the size of a pea in the brain, which controls the production of several hormones. From puberty onwards these four hormones play their part in regulating the menstrual cycle.

Each follows its own pattern, rising and falling at different points in the cycle, but together they produce a predictable chain of events. One egg (out of thousands in each ovary) becomes 'ripe' (mature) and is released from one of the ovaries. As the egg starts its journey down the Fallopian tube to the womb, the ovaries switch to producing progesterone, which encourages the blood supply to the womb lining (the endometrium) in case it is called up to nourish a growing *embryo* (what the egg is called once fertilized). If the egg isn't fertilized, the levels of oestrogen and progesterone produced by the ovary begin to fall. Without the supporting action of these hormones, the womb lining, which is full of blood, is shed, resulting in a period.

At this point the levels of both progesterone and oestrogen are at their lowest level in the body. The brain registers this and sends signals to the pituitary gland to step up production of FSH, and the whole cycle starts again.

A woman has a finite number of eggs and her ovaries can only carry on releasing them for a finite amount of time. From her thirties onwards she may not ovulate during every monthly period, which upsets the normal balance of her hormones. Without ovulation the ovaries do not step up production of progesterone. Failure to ovulate also prompts the brain to call for more FSH, which will in turn stimulate the ovaries to step up oestrogen production and go into overdrive, so the woman will experience a sort of oestrogen-overload. Unopposed by progesterone, the cell-stimulating effect of oestrogen (strictly speaking, oestradiol) will increase the risk of cancer of the endometrium. Hormonal imbalance is the most likely cause of the heavy and irregular bleeding at the menopause. Ultimately, of course, the ovaries pack up egg and hormone production and the levels in the blood plummet. The menopause has brought fertility to a stop.

'Gosh, it's hot in here'

The hot flush (hot flash in the USA), or night sweat is one of the most distinctive symptoms of the menopause. In the West three-quarters or more of women going through the menopause say they have them. (Interesting cultural variations are discussed in the next chapter.) Untreated, they may last for at least five years or more. In crude terms these are caused by the ovaries cutting back production of oestradiol – the strong, premenopausal type of oestrogen. This is demonstrated by the fact that giving a woman pharmaceutically manufactured oestrogens immediately stops the hot flushes. If asked, doctors will usually tell you that shortage of oestrogen affects the body's heat-regulating mechanism, though it is a bit more complicated than that. If you can take a little more science see the box *Body thermostat malfunctions.*

Body thermostat malfunctions

Researchers at Wayne State University in Detroit (USA) have dedicated a lifetime to studying the hot flush and they have discovered what you might have imagined, knowing about hormones and emotions – that hot flushes are not just a physical thing, experienced in the body, they have a psychological dimension. Changes were discovered in a particular part of the brain in menopausal women experiencing a hot flush that didn't occur in the brains of women who were made hot and sweaty by being surrounded with hot pads: the part of the brain concerned with perceiving temperature, pain, hunger and erotic experiences. The body has a sort of thermostat that regulates temperature so that if it gets too hot you start to sweat, if too cold you begin to shiver. In between these two extremes that prompt a physical response is a neutral area. The Wayne researchers found that the women with the most intense hot flushes had a very narrow or non-existent neutral zone. Apparently the size of the neutral zone – in other words, the temperature at which someone starts to perspire – is affected by another hormone that you may have heard of, *noradrenaline* (norepinephrine in the USA), sometimes known as the stress hormone because it gees the body up to fight or flee when threatened. This might explain why a hot flush is also often accompanied by a pounding heart or a surge of panic. These emotions when experienced in response to a genuine threat can also make you experience a momentary hot flush. Noradrenaline is known to act on the part of the brain that regulates the body's thermostat, so the hypothesis is that a drop in oestrogen levels sends a message to the brain causing it to release noradrenaline, setting off the chain of events that leads to a hot flush. In animal experiments an increase of noradrenaline in the brain lowered the level at which they started to perspire. To test this hypothesis the Wayne researchers heated up two groups of menopausal women, one on HRT (taking artificial oestrogen) and one without, and discovered that the women on HRT remained cool at a higher temperature than those not taking it.

And another thing ...

We have taken a fair amount of space to cover just two symptoms of the menopause – mood swings and hot flushes. This is because in discussing them we have taken on board the complex inter-relation between various hormones that control not only fertility but many other physical, mental and emotional processes as well as a woman's monthly periods. When we come to consider the full range of symptoms recorded by women during and after the menopause we find that many of them can be traced to the same changes – fluctuating or failing hormones. These can explain the sleep problems, headaches, heart flutters and fatigue often reported. In the case of the latter yet another hormone may be implicated: low testosterone – a hormone more significant in men but which affects energy levels and libido in both sexes. Loss of oestrogen is thought to be behind vaginal dryness – oestrogen plumped up and lubricated this important channel at puberty, and, as it tails off, the vagina shrinks and becomes drier which can lead to uncomfortable sexual intercourse unless a substitute lubricant is used. Some sources list wrinkles and changes in hair quality as symptoms of the menopause, but here we come up against the fact that these things happen to men also and are inevitably part of the business of growing older. Weight gain, or more specifically, new fat deposits – around the middle, on the back and upper arms – also tends to occur at around this time, though how much this is to do with hormone levels is not clear.

Meanwhile, *after* the menopause

We have concentrated in this chapter on the symptoms that occur before (the *perimenopause*) and during the menopause. This is how you will encounter the event. But I have also tried to explain that the hormonal changes that occur now do not just affect fertility, mood, heat regulation and the quality of the skin. These important body chemicals operate on many body systems and lead to changes that are not just temporary but long-lasting and, in many ways, more serious. In later chapters we will look at the important effects of passing the menopause on bone density, your heart and blood vessels, bladder, brain, breasts, womb and vagina, and other parts of the body, as well as how to take all these changes in your stride, keep healthy and still have fun.

2

Natural event or historic accident?

So what's so special about the menopause? We don't get so steamed up about the menarche, when periods start. Men are only now getting a little attention for their 'mid-life crisis', which was recently rechristened the 'andropause' (*andro* being a Greek word for man). The most obvious explanation is that in the past not enough women lived long enough to reach the menopause for it to be seen as a significant event. In the seventeenth century less than a third of women lived to experience the menopause. At the industrial revolution, average life expectancy in the cities, even among the gentry, was less than 40 years, and among the urban working class was at most 20. Even in the countryside not many women made it to 50. If you didn't die in pregnancy or childbirth, you were as likely to succumb to tuberculosis or to one of the epidemics of cholera or typhus that were a standard hazard of life then. No wonder that the event didn't even get a proper name until the early nineteenth century.

Menopause long ago and far away

Nevertheless, as the Bible records, the natural human lifespan (the age someone lived to if not struck down by war, famine or pestilence) has, since that time, been relatively constant at 'three score years and ten'. Since antiquity a percentage of women have lived to experience life after the menopause and no man could fail to have observed it. The ancient Greek philosopher Aristotle notes the event as occurring then, as now the world over, somewhere between the fifth and sixth decade. The medieval physician Galen recommended bleeding, so that any 'retained poisons' could be released. (Mind you, in those days they thought bleeding a treatment for everything, including anaemia.) In the sixteenth century purgatives and the application of leeches were popular – again for a wide range of medical conditions. In 1777 John Leake recommends a modified diet: 'Where the patient is delicate and subject to female weakness, night sweats or an habitual purging, with flushing in the face and a hectic fever: for such; ass's milk, jellies and raw eggs, with cooling fruits. At meals she may be indulged with half a pint of old, clear London porter, or a glass of Rhenish wine.'

The menopause is acknowledged as a natural event; but is it a medical condition – requiring treatment? The Canadian anthropologist Joel Wilbrush dates the medicalization of the menopause to the French Revolution. The word itself was coined in 1816 by a French physician, de Gardanne: 'la menespausie', later modified to 'menopause', from the Greek for month (*men*) and cessation (*pausis*). Wilbrush writes, 'No menopausal disturbances are however recorded until the social convulsions of the French Revolution, and the regimes which followed, seem to have crystallised the various complaints of the climacteric [another word for the menopause] into a disease-expression, which reified [made concrete] the social stress to which women were subject.' This is a familiar theme in feminist writing today.

All was not bad news for menopausal women in antiquity. Although it is not exhaustively chronicled, there is evidence that some societies in ancient China, India and among the North American Indians revered women who survived beyond their childbearing years. Women in these societies were symbols of fertility and growth and the old were respected and valued as a source of wisdom. The postmenopausal woman was regarded as uniquely qualified to support younger women through pregnancy and childbirth.

This positive view of the menopause informs the modern idea that the menopause may actually be an evolutionary adaptation among human beings; what has come to be known as the 'caring grandmother' hypothesis.

Why menopause?

There are two major theories as to why the human female should cease to be fertile such a long time before she hangs up her boots. The first is that giving birth is a risky business and the older you are the more it is likely to kill you, so that a woman who stops getting pregnant at 50 will still have time to raise her last child. Human children are dependent for much longer than other young mammals; it therefore requires approaching 16 years following the menopause (near enough to the natural human lifespan) to guarantee this. This idea is supported by research on social mammals – lions and baboons for example – who become infertile just long enough to support their last infant before the end of their natural lifespan (see box: *Lions do it, baboons do it*).

Lions do it, baboons do it

In an article called 'Why menopause?' in *Natural History Magazine* in 1998, Craig Packer, professor in the Department of Ecology, Evolution, and Behavior at the University of Michigan, USA, argued elegantly against the 'caring grandmother' hypothesis of the menopause, quoting evidence from his long-term studies of two species often viewed as useful models of the evolution in man: the olive baboon and the African lion. These species live in complex social groups that revolve around the relationships of female kin. In the lion pride a core of female relatives hunt, defend a joint territory, and raise cubs communally – to the extent not just of 'babysitting' but even suckling one another's young. Baboons form family-based social groups, with a clear pecking order in which daughters rank just below their mothers. Elderly females frequently groom and care for their grandchildren.

As Packer notes, few animals in the wild live to old age, but lions, exceptionally, are seldom attacked by other species and often survive into their dotage. They were able, over several decades, to estimate the lion's natural lifespan as 18 years. By 17 a lioness's reproductive days were over, which left her with approximately a year of natural lifespan: almost exactly the time it takes for a lion-cub to become capable of surviving without her. There is a similar pattern in baboons: they start reproducing at six; their fertility declines over the years; by the time they reach 27 their menstrual cycle ceases altogether; and no baboon lives to be more than 28: just long enough to rear her last-born infant.

Clearly granny lionesses and baboons do not stop having young to devote themselves to their daughters' offspring. The 'grandchildren' survived just as well when granny was dead as when she was alive and postmenopausal. In fact Packer found that with lions a grandmother only improved the survival odds of her grandchildren when she continued to bear young herself, since she could only suckle cubs if she had produced her own litter. An end to cub-bearing was an end to her ability to look after her grand-cubs too.

Packer concludes: 'Studies like ours suggest that menopause is not only a universal feature of mammalian life history but also an inevitable legacy of the very feature that defines mammals: the remarkable care that we receive from our mothers.'

The 'caring grandmother' theory may not receive support from a study of lions and baboons, but what about humans? Two recent studies, looking at people living in African villages where life approximated to how it might have been for our hunter-gather forefathers, were reported in the *Proceedings of the Royal Society* in 2007. These found that human grandmothers did indeed improve the chance of survival among their grandchildren. If a child's mother died before it was two years old its chance of survival to adulthood fell by 10 per cent. But if its maternal grandmother was still alive this reduction was cut to only 5 per cent. No other relative had any effect on a child's survival. The team concluded that caring grannies conferred an evolutionary advantage: they would help a population expand.

However, not all primitive people regard the postmenopausal grandmother as an unalloyed blessing. Some nomadic South American tribes traditionally abandon grandmothers, possibly because there is not enough food to go round, and those that survive do nothing to improve the survival of their grandchildren. Although the postmenopausal grannies had marginally more children than those who died before they reached 50, they actually had fewer grandchildren – by as much as 50 per cent. The researchers argued that although women living to a great age might improve the survival chances of their *own* children by being good mothers, having these grannies around created a strain on resources that actually harmed their daughters' children. These conflicting results were explained by researchers with the hypothesis that in South America, in the past, grandmothers did little to help their daughters, whereas among the African groups studied they did, and by so doing improved the odds on their grandchildren's survival.

These days, fortunately, there are fewer environments where a woman living past the menopause might be a drain on scarce resources. In fact in developed countries the birth rate has dropped so far that it is grandchildren who are in short supply, leading to competition between grandmothers over who shall help look after them. And since those postmenopausal women who do have grandchildren are just as likely to have careers that keep them fully occupied, or interesting social lives that take them all over the place, rather than spending their time knitting in a rocking chair waiting to babysit, they are probably not as worried about *why* they should be going through the menopause as about how best to survive it.

Attitudes to the menopause and its treatment

Women who are not anthropologists may not worry much about the role of the menopause in evolution. Nevertheless, social attitudes affect how they experience the event, and also how doctors respond to it, and these things vary; throughout history, in different cultures and among different ethnic groups. A Study of Women's Health Across the Nation (SWAN), ongoing in the United States, discovered big differences in reported menopausal symptoms among women from different ethnic backgrounds. There isn't even a word for hot flushes in some languages, the study says. SWAN found that nearly 50 per cent of Latin American women reported hot flushes (flashes); slightly fewer African Americans, followed by the Japanese, with just under 30 per cent of European-descent women reporting them, and the lowest incidence of all among Chinese women. Latin American women seemed to suffer most from a number of other menopausal symptoms like painful intercourse, vaginal infection and sleep disturbance, closely followed by African Americans, and with the lowest number of Asian women reporting such symptoms.

Attitudes to the menopause vary widely within Europe also, and these conflicting attitudes may partly explain why women react differently when the menopause hits them. At one extreme are those that see it is a simple biological event – nature taking its course; what are you making such a fuss about? At the other end it is viewed as an illness, a 'condition', rather as the Victorians used to talk about pregnancy being an 'interesting condition'. In fact all the mysteries of a woman's fertile body – menstruation, childbirth and the menopause – are sometimes spoken of as something to be treated: the illness of being a woman.

In the sixteenth and seventeenth centuries physicians treated the cessation of periods with whatever therapy was in vogue at the time. Since at that time illnesses were attributed to evil 'humours', or body fluids, they treated the menopause, along with other conditions, with leeches, purges, blood-letting or plant extracts known to cause menstrual bleeding. In the nineteenth century doctors sought explanations in particular organs of the body, and since women were distinguished by the possession of a womb and a pair of ovaries, those unfortunate organs were blamed for a vast range of physiological or psychological conditions thought to be particular to women, and they were treated by removal of the organs. Of course, if you take out the ovaries you cut off the supply of oestradiol and a woman goes through an artificial early menopause. (These days, if ovaries need to be removed because of disease, wherever possible surgeons will go to great lengths to leave a tiny piece of one ovary in place simply to continue the hormonal cycle and avoid causing an early menopause.)

Hormones identified

We now know that the menstrual cycle, along with many other physical processes, is controlled by the subtle interaction between several hormones. But the existence of these mysterious, naturally occurring chemicals, which affect several different physical systems throughout the body including mood, was discovered by accident. In 1889 a 72-year-old French doctor called Brown-Séquard published a paper in the *Lancet* claiming to have experienced a dramatic resurgence of youthful vitality after injecting himself with extracts from guinea pig and dog testicles. The report led to the widespread use of testicular extracts, which contain the important male hormone now known as *testosterone*, to counter the effects of ageing. Brown-Séquard also suggested that an ovarian extract might have a rejuvenating effect on women. Two German doctors treating a young woman for hot flushes following the removal of her ovaries were the first to put this theory to the test. They fed her ground-up animal ovaries. It didn't help, but at least it didn't kill her. More than 30 years later a researcher called Serge Voronoff conducted some scarily crude hormone therapy experiments that involved grafting monkey ovaries into women, and actually killed some of them – the women as well as the monkeys. Although scientists had become aware of hormones, they hadn't yet discovered about rejection – the mechanism by which the body recognizes any foreign biological material and destroys it.

In the years that followed one important hormone after another was identified, but the various forms of oestrogen continued to fox the researchers. Finally, at the end of the 1920s, different teams of researchers in the USA and in Germany succeeded in isolating one form of the hormone, which was given a number of names before being called oestrogen (estrogen in the USA). The first drug to treat the menopause, based on this, and extracted from the urine of pregnant women, became available in 1930. Supply was still limited because it was difficult to produce, and it wasn't until it was discovered that oestrogen could also be isolated from the urine of pregnant mares, in 1943, that an effective form of replacement oestrogen was marketed under a name still in use to day – Premarin.

'Forever feminine'

You will notice that there is no mention of progesterone at this stage, or any attempt to design hormone replacement that would mimic the complex interaction of the different hormones that control the natural menstrual cycle. Oestrogen on its own – unopposed oestrogen as it is called – certainly sorted out those troublesome hot flushes and boosted mood and energy levels, but it carried in its wake a chain of negative side effects. Doctors remained unconvinced. So the company behind Premarin launched a massive effort to 'educate' doctors about the drug. It was greatly aided by a New York gynaecologist called Robert Wilson, who published first a paper in a respected medical journal and later a book called *Forever Feminine*, in which he described the menopause as 'nature's defeminization' and blamed loss of oestrogen for a range of health problems including osteoporosis. By emphasizing oestrogen's beneficial effect on bone health, a known problem for postmenopausal women, Wilson captured the attention of his colleagues, but he went further. He painted a dramatic picture of women going through the menopause as emotionally disturbed, sick, exhausted, dried up and deprived of their femininity. He invented a 'preventable' illness which he called 'oestrogen deficiency disease', which would be 'cured' by taking hormone replacement. He went so far as to describe loss of functional ovaries as 'female castration'.

It was good news in that it encouraged doctors to acknowledge that for a fair number of women, going through the menopause was no bed of roses. And Wilson published his book in 1966, at a time when feminism was first starting to flex its muscles in America and Europe. Wilson's crusade seemed to promise women a vigorous, healthy life after the menopause, something feminists welcomed. But it also cast what was essentially a natural biological event as the death of femininity, as though women were defined purely by the activity of their ovaries; not so different from previous generations who had defined them in terms of their roles as wives and mothers. As such, his message was definitely regressive and feminists deplored it. Basically he was saying, in the words of the old popular song, 'look young and beautiful if you want to be loved'.

Hormones opposed

But in promoting oestrogen as some kind of elixir of youth, Wilson spoke directly to women facing middle age at a time when there had never been more emphasis on youth. By 1975 Premarin had become one of the most widely prescribed medicines in the western world. And then came the bad news. Studies were published showing that oestrogen (remember it was oestrogen on its own that women were taking then) increased cancer of the lining of the womb. Doctors and patients panicked: the one stopped prescribing, the other stopped taking the pills. Sales plummeted. But within a few years, in 1980, the drug manufacturers came up with a new formula that approximated more closely to the natural menstrual cycle. Women took oestrogen for three weeks of their cycle, then swapped it for a form of progesterone called *progestogen*, and the withdrawal caused the womb lining (endometrium) to come away in a bleed that resembled a normal period. Natural progesterone prepares the womb lining for pregnancy, and the manufactured version of it is also protective against cancer. It is this 'combined' hormone replacement that is understood when people talk about HRT – hormone replacement therapy.

Later in the book we look at the pros and cons of HRT and whether taking it is right for you. Here we are more interested in looking at how medical and social attitudes affect the way the menopause is treated. In the twenty-first century women in the West have lives that extend well beyond marriage and motherhood. Even their fertile years may not be entirely devoted to having children, and they may live for a further 40 years when this is no longer an option. In abandoning widows' weeds and rocking chairs, modern women of 50 have also been challenged by the possibility that they might also give up the menopause and hold on to their hormones. It is their choice, but it is also in some ways a poisoned chalice.

There are signs that the attitudes of the societies in which we live still affect this choice, and also how women experience the change of life. In the West it's sometimes possible to get the feeling that staying young and attractive is just a matter of effort and dedication. Only backsliders who don't diet or exercise get old. This may go some way to explain why, even today, more western women have a worse time during the menopause than Asian women, whose society regards old age as something dignified, to be respected.

3

When menopause?

The average age for a woman living in the UK in the twenty-first century to go through the menopause is 52 years. This age appears to have remained remarkably consistent throughout time (Aristotle, in ancient Greece, notes it occurring some time between the fifth and sixth decade) and throughout the globe. Nevertheless, although small, there are variations between individual women. A number of factors contribute to these differences.

- About 85 per cent of the variation is almost certainly a matter of genes. According to a Dutch study of 243 sisters from 118 families, women in the same family go through the menopause at about the same age. So do women from the same ethnic group. Studies of women from different ethnic groups living in America revealed that Japanese women tended to have a slightly later menopause and Latin Americans a slighter earlier one, than women of European origin.
- Poor nutrition may play a part. Women who were small as babies or malnourished as children tend to have an early menopause. So do women with a low body mass index – in other words, who are thin.
- Several studies implicate cigarette smoking. Norwegian research on more than 2,000 women found that smokers were more than 59 per cent more likely to go through the menopause before 45 than non-smokers.
- A recent massive Polish study of more than 7,000 women discovered other factors: starting the periods early, having a menstrual cycle of short duration, a low level of educational achievement, having a 'negative health perception', as well as smoking cigarettes. The same study found that having had children or taken oral contraceptives were associated with a later than average menopause.

- The season of your birth may also make a difference. An Italian study of more than 3,000 women found that spring-born women tended to experience the menopause on average a year earlier than the autumn-born, though the researchers provided no explanation for the effect. An amazing number of things, from suicide to autism, seem to have season of birth variations. Theories as to why this should be vary, but the effect of sunshine hours, and maternal nutrition on the baby in the womb have been suggested. (It's probably not the influence of the stars.)

These small variations in the age of the natural menopause are probably only important to a woman hoping to have children later in life. But there are other more serious causes of an early menopause: illness and surgery.

Premature menopause or premature ovarian failure (POF)

There is a clear distinction between early menopause and premature menopause, otherwise known more precisely as premature ovarian failure (POF). The first is just part of the normal variation in a natural biological event. The latter is a result either of illness or a medical condition, or a consequence of treatment for some medical condition. If you have to have both ovaries removed (a bilateral *oophorectomy*), or if you have both ovaries, the womb and both Fallopian tubes removed (a total *hysterectomy*), your oestrogen and progesterone levels will immediately plunge, throwing you into a sudden and immediate menopause. Wherever possible, surgeons who need to operate on these organs leave just a small piece of one ovary in place, in order to maintain a normal cycle afterwards, but there are occasions when this is not possible. When this happens a woman may experience more intense symptoms than those simply going through an early menopause, because instead of tailing off gradually their hormonal cycle is cut off abruptly, in its prime. When this happens, treating the symptoms of the premature menopause is an integral part of the aftercare of surgery.

There are other forms of surgery that may accidentally damage the ovaries. Sometimes after a hysterectomy, one in which the surgeon has left one, or even both ovaries intact, one or both may fail, either immediately after the operation or up to a few years later. The ovaries can become damaged when a *cyst* (a small sac filled with fluid) is removed, or if the surgeon accidentally damages blood vessels carrying blood to the ovaries. When this happens the remaining *follicles* on the ovary/ovaries slowly die out, bringing on the menopause. Having your 'tubes tied' – what is known medically as *tubal ligation*, or sterilization – also occasionally interferes with the blood flow to the ovaries, leading eventually to POF.

In addition to surgery, drugs, chemotherapy and radiation therapy to treat some forms of cancer may also cause the ovaries to fail. Low-dose/short-term treatment may simply interrupt the normal function, and a normal cycle may then resume after a few months, but often, even if the periods start again, the woman may be left infertile. The drug Tamoxifen is extremely effective in the treatment of breast cancer and cuts breast cancer rates by about 45 per cent. But it locks on to receptors in the body that normally react to oestrogen, thereby preventing oestrogen performing its usual role in the menstrual cycle, and causing POF. Fortunately

Restoring fertility after cancer treatment

There are highly successful ways of freezing a fertilized egg outside a woman's body if she is about to undergo cancer treatment that could make her infertile. The egg can then be replanted in the womb, and she may become pregnant once the treatment is complete. However, it is much more difficult to freeze/preserve unfertilized female ova for a woman without a partner to provide sperm for fertilization. There have been a number of successful animal experiments, in Israel with sheep, and in Japan with monkeys, where female ovaries have been successfully removed, frozen and then later returned to the donor where they have been able to establish normal hormone production. One or two US medical centres are now offering this service to young women compelled to undergo cancer treatment. The ovary is removed, the tissue carefully dissected with microsurgery, frozen, and subsequently transplanted back to the woman after she has been cured of the cancer. Theoretically this treatment might also be offered to women wishing to conceive later in life, when the quality of their ova is poorer. Although no successful pregnancies have yet been reported, it is probably only a matter of time.

this effect is sometimes only temporary and the normal pattern of fertility resumes once treatment stops. Other drugs that may interrupt the normal cycle and bring on a temporary menopause are those prescribed to treat two common conditions that cause painful, heavy periods: *endometriosis* (where the type of tissue that lines the womb develops in other parts of the body, for example the ovaries), and drugs to shrink uterine fibroids – non-cancerous growths that develop in the muscular wall of the womb – prior to removing them surgically.

One other quite common cause of POF is a disorder of the *autoimmune system*. Some recent studies suggest that more than 60 per cent of women whose ovaries shut down prematurely do so because the body's immune system mistakenly attacks the body itself. It's as though the body suddenly identifies part of itself as an invader and sends out antibodies to destroy this perceived threat. In the case of POF women may develop antibodies to their own ovarian tissue, to the endometrium or to one or more of the hormones that regulate ovulation, and this causes the whole reproductive cycle to shut down. Women with a family history of autoimmune disorders such as thyroid disease, diabetes, or rheumatoid arthritis, may be more prone to this type of early menopause.

There are several less common causes of POF. Some infections, fortunately rare in developed countries, can temporarily or even permanently stop the ovaries working. These include tuberculosis (TB), malaria, mumps and chickenpox. Most children are vaccinated against the last two these days. Some experts also think that environmental toxins – substances like the agro-chemical DDT or chemicals in other pesticides, cleaning products, cosmetics, food additives, drugs, and common or garden plastic containers used to store and prepare food, all of which have been used in increasing quantities in recent years, and the majority of which have not been tested for human safety – could be affecting the hormone levels in both sexes, thereby increasing the incidence of premature menopause.

If for some reason you are facing an early or premature menopause you can find a wealth of helpful information on the website <www.earlymenopause.com/>. For women distressed by the situation and still wishing to become pregnant, there is the possibility of *in vitro fertilization* (IVF) using donor eggs. There is a UK support organization called the Daisy Network which will help you discuss the options, and there is also International Premature Ovarian Failure Association.

Are there tests for the menopause?

In books about an illness a chapter will usually be devoted to diagnosis; symptoms apart, how do the doctors work out what you are suffering from? The menopause is, we need hardly repeat, *not* an illness, nor is it necessary to do tests to prove that it is taking place. Nevertheless there are situations, like experiencing an early menopause, when you may be asked to undergo some tests to check what is going on in your body; there are also tests it is advisable to take to check your health, both before and after this time. Some screening tests you may already be familiar with because women are recommended to start them before the menopause.

You may sail through your later years without the need for any of these tests. Nevertheless the health conditions they test for become more significant as you get older and some of them are more important if you decide to take HRT, so it is as well to become familiar with them.

Cervical smear

All women between the ages of 25 and 64 are advised to undergo screening for changes in the cells of the neck of the womb (*cervix*) that warn of possible cancer. A smear can be taken in the GP's surgery and involves taking a small sample of cells from the neck of the womb and sending them for analysis in the laboratory. If early changes in these cells are detected, treatment can prevent cancer developing.

Breast screening

Women in high-risk groups (having a family history of breast cancer and/or carrying one of the known breast-cancer genes) are usually encouraged to have a *mammogram* from the age of 40. From the ages of 50 to 70 (soon to be extended to 47 to 73) women in England are invited to have a scan once every three years. It involves squashing the breast onto a low-dose X-ray machine (some people find it uncomfortable, but it doesn't really hurt) and taking images that reveal any small changes in the cells of the breast that may indicate the warning signs of cancer. Some types of HRT affect the way the breast tissue appears on a mammogram, although oestrogen on its own does not seem to cause these changes. You may also be encouraged to examine your breasts yourself, although there is little evidence that woman are as good at detecting something abnormal as an X-ray machine.

Hormone tests

As we have already explained, there are several different hormones involved in controlling the normal menstrual cycle, and measuring the levels present in the body can indicate either that the menopause has started or that some other condition is responsible for the symptoms. Tests are often done to rule things out as well as rule things in. At different ages your doctor may take a sample of blood to test for levels of different hormones circulating in your body. Women younger than 45 may be tested for levels of follicle-stimulating hormone (FSH) if their doctor is unsure whether they are going through an early menopause. A test for *thyroid* function may also be made because this hormone is responsible for heat regulation, among other things, and a thyroid problem may be confused with menopausal symptoms. Women taking HRT but not responding well may be asked to have a test to discover what levels of oestradiol, from an implant, patch or gel, are actually finding their way into the blood stream.

Examining the lining of the womb

Checking the cells that line the womb is very important for problems like fibroids, heavy bleeding and for women taking HRT. The first test is usually an *ultrasound* scan – a picture built up by bouncing sound waves off the different tissue in the body. It is done in hospital, but without anaesthetics, usually by sliding the ultrasound probe over the stomach above the womb, but sometimes via the vagina. It enables the experts to judge how thick the endometrial lining is, and to check for fibroids or cysts.

Biopsy

Sometimes a sample of cells may be taken from the womb lining, rather as they are from the cervix during a smear, in order to put them under the microscope in the laboratory and check for abnormalities. This is usually done, without anaesthetic, by passing a fine tube up through the cervix into the womb and gently sucking up a few cells from the endometrium.

Hysteroscopy

This procedure also involves passing a fine tube through the cervix and into the womb, but this time it is equipped with a telescope so that the surface of the endometrium can be viewed by the doctor doing the examination. Hysteroscopy and biopsy are often done at the same time if abnormalities detected on the ultrasound scan require further investigation. Both can be done without anaesthetic, with local anaesthetic, or in hospital under a general anaesthetic. It depends on a number of factors including how flexible the neck of the womb is.

Bone density scans

If you have a family history of osteoporosis (brittle bones) you may have an X-ray bone density scan even before you reach the menopause. Most healthy women do not require a scan even after the menopause. However, since there is a risk of osteoporosis the older you get, your GP may decide it would be wise to check for it. The gold-standard bone density scan is called *dual-energy X-ray absorbtiometry* (DEXA) – the different energies distinguish between soft tissue and bone – and it accurately measures the mineral density of bone. It is usually carried out on the hip or spine. Single density X-ray absorbtiometry may be used for wrist scans but is not as accurate as hip and spine measurements. Other tests, not using X-rays, are also being developed. Ultrasound may be able to test the strength of the bone of the heel, and it may ultimately be possible to diagnose osteoporosis from a blood or urine test by measuring a number of chemicals found in the blood that are associated with the build-up and breakdown of bone.

4

Do we, don't we, treat the menopause?

You rush home from the supermarket, sweat soaking your shirt and trickling down your neck, and throw yourself under a cold shower – and it's midwinter; two degrees above zero. You break away from your husband's tender advances because intercourse has become agony. Driving, you are seized by sudden panic at the sight of a car waiting to pull out of a side street ahead of you; you feel dizzy, sick with apprehension and your heart thumps in your chest. The car ahead waits patiently for you to pass.

These are symptoms familiar to women who have been through the menopause. In addition to the much-quoted hot flushes (flashes in the USA) sometimes followed by the shivers, the painful intercourse caused by the thinning and drying out of the lining of the vagina, the disturbed sleep, sudden palpitations and anxiety attacks, caused by hormonal disturbance, here are some well-documented others.

- Irregular periods
- *Hypoglycaemia* (low blood sugar): suddenly feeling weak or shaky, slightly sick and breaking out in a cold sweat
- Disturbed gut: bloating, indigestion, painful stomach gas or flatulence, diarrhoea, constipation
- *Cystitis* (infections of the urinary system)
- Breast tenderness
- Cold hands and feet
- Joint pain
- Mood changes
- Forgetfulness, inability to concentrate.

We make no apology for returning to the place where we started: to the symptoms that women experience when they hit the menopause. These symptoms are a woman's first introduction to the whole topic. In Chapter 1 we drew a distinction between the short-term and the long-term symptoms, both caused by a drop in hormone production but leading to knock-on effects throughout the body. The short-term symptoms that announce and characterize the change are uncomfortable, but are over in a matter of a few years. The long-term changes that develop after the menopause are in many ways more serious since they can have major effects on your health. Later in the book (Chapters 6 to 9) we look at how a drop in hormone levels influences systems throughout the body: the heart and circulation, its susceptibility to cancer, bone density, skin, brain and the urinary system. Sorting these changes from the inevitable passage of the years is pretty difficult, although the widespread use of HRT has made this a little easier in recent years.

But let's start with the early symptoms listed above and what can be done to relieve them. It might seem obvious that since this experience affects all women who reach a certain age, and since a vast number of them have the same symptoms, many of them unpleasant and debilitating, that all hands would be joined to treat these symptoms. Sadly that has not been the case. This is partly because it wasn't until the turn of the twentieth century that doctors had some idea of *why* a woman's periods stopped, let alone what health problems were heralded by the change. Early attempts to treat the symptoms were therefore almost inevitably rather hit and miss. 'Ass's milk, jellies and raw eggs, with cooling fruits ... half a pint of old, clear London porter, or a glass of Rhenish wine,' being among the more acceptable early remedies on offer.

Meddling with nature

But ignorance of the underlying cause was just one obstacle. For many years treating the menopause also came up against a problem that has bedevilled treating other 'women's conditions', like painful periods (*dysmenorrhoea*), infertility, labour or unwanted pregnancy. These events were all considered 'natural', hence God-given. Deep in the social (and medical) unconscious is a fear of 'meddling with nature'. You hear the same concern where food is concerned, or sexual behaviour. What is natural equals what is good. And what is 'natural' often gets equated with 'what has always happened'. The fact that human beings have colonized the earth chiefly by manipulating what comes naturally, particularly when it comes to what makes life more comfortable and last longer, gets ignored. Death also is a natural event, but most of us are happy to put it off by every means at our disposal.

There was the most frightful resistance to administering anaesthetics to ease childbirth until Queen Victoria provided a lead and took chloroform at the birth of her eighth child, Prince Leopold. Women were *supposed* to suffer in childbirth; it says so in the Bible. In my own lifetime there was fierce resistance to the use of birth control or the termination of pregnancy (religious faith quite apart). Preventing or terminating pregnancy, or artificially aiding it, ruffles a lot of moral and religious feathers. And there was, and still is, a resistance to treating the menopause that is much broader and deeper than the reasonable concerns about the side effects of HRT – most of which were discovered somewhat later than the drugs themselves and offered convenient legitimization to an irrational resistance to the use of 'artificial' hormones.

Doctors are always a little uncomfortable when expected to treat anything other than what they recognize as disorder or malfunction. What they call the 'medical model' is a version of 'if it ain't broke, don't fix it'. Doctors know what their goals are if they are faced with something that is not working properly. Trying to prescribe something to make us healthy, or to modify normal bodily functions like having babies or not, or having periods or not, in order to improve the quality of life, takes them into territory sometimes known as 'lifestyle' choices. So perhaps it is to some extent fortunate that the discovery that there were serious, long-term physical consequences of going through the menopause – brittle bones (*osteoporosis*) and a higher risk of coronary artery disease – made addressing these problems a distinct medical priority. Hot flushes, moods and painful intercourse might be regarded as tough luck, but just the way the cookie crumbles for our unfortunate sex. Increased risk of hip fractures and heart attack is real illness, unlike limiting fertility or aiding it artificially. Treating these risks is clearly important.

In fact, I strongly suspect that if HRT hadn't got itself labelled a 'youth elixir' the medical profession would have found it a great deal more acceptable. As it is, since it first made its appearance 70 or 80 years ago opinion has been divided, and there has been a repeated swing of the pendulum either way in favour or against it, and the see-saw has left the profession noticeably divided.

HRT and your personal health profile

Tara Parker Pope, in her book *HRT: Everything you need to know*, charts the pendulum swings in the popularity chart of the treatment in admirably explained detail. In the next chapter I will return to this in trying to help you make sense of the many ongoing scientific studies of postmenopausal health and the effect of HRT upon it and their sometimes conflicting findings, and finally decide if it is for you or not. The menopause is life-changing but not life-threatening, so ultimately whether you treat the short-term discomforts or the long-term health risks is a matter of personal choice that depends upon your priorities as well as your individual risk profile.

There is, of course, one aspect of the menopause that can not be treated. Nothing can restore your ovaries' natural egg production. The menopause occurs because all the follicles capable of developing eggs in your ovaries have run out. They have been falling by the wayside steadily since you were conceived. It's possible that a way to slow down this extravagant wastefulness may one day be discovered, but women currently have at least 30 years in which to have babies and there are plenty of other satisfying things to do in the last decades of their lives.

Drug treatments for the menopause

Since the unpleasant symptoms of the menopause are caused by a fall in levels of oestrogen produced in the body it is no surprise to find that replacing this supply with similar hormones, produced in the laboratory, cures or alleviates many of them. However, as I explained in Chapter 2, if you still have your womb, unopposed oestrogen can harm the lining (endometrium). A second replacement hormone called progestogen, protective of the womb lining, is added to modern HRT. These two hormones mimic the action of naturally produced hormones, but have been engineered and

What's in HRT?

In Chapter 2 we recounted how, in the 1920s, doctors discovered how to extract a hormone, ultimately named oestrogen, from the urine of pregnant women, and later from pregnant mares. This became the first replacement hormone used to treat the symptoms of the menopause. These days other forms of the oestrogen have been isolated from soya beans and yams, but the form of oestrogen obtained from pregnant mares is still an important source. These *equine* oestrogens contain between 50 and 65 per cent oestrone sulphate, which is the same as the human form, although the remainder are animal oestrogens. Totally synthetic oestrogens are also manufactured in the laboratory and used in the contraceptive pill. These have a much more powerful effect on the body and are not suitable for treating menopausal symptoms. The form of oestrogen used in contemporary HRT is oestradiol.

The other hormone in HRT is progestogen. This is not there to treat symptoms but to protect against the side effects of unopposed oestrogen. The natural form of this hormone is called progesterone. The form used in HRT derives mostly from plant sources such as yams. There are two sorts of progestogens: those very like progesterone and those based on testosterone, another hormone, but active in both sexes. The latter can give rise to side effects of their own such as mood swings, depression, headaches and breast tenderness. There is a third, newer form of progestogen, slightly closer to natural progesterone, called *drospirenone*, which has previously been used for contraceptive pills and was introduced in the USA in 2007 as a form of HRT called Angeliq.

You will encounter the distinction 'natural' and 'synthetic' applied to the hormones in HRT. This is a bit confusing because none of these compounds is identical to what the body produces. Some, like the equine oestrogen referred to above which is the basis of the oldest of HRT drugs, Premarin or Prempak-C, are closer to natural oestrogen than others. Tablets that contain oestradiol, oestriol, and oestrone are often called 'natural' oestrogens because they either contain forms of oestrogen that are produced naturally in a woman's body, or are converted into these forms in the body before they enter the bloodstream. In this book I use natural (without quote marks) only when I discuss what is made by the human body. Synthetic hormones are stronger than the so-called natural ones and are mainly used for contraceptives.

tested by a pharmaceutical company. You may hear such drugs compared unfavourably, not only to the 'natural' hormones made by the human body but also to hormones derived from vegetables – herbal preparations. There are a number of plant preparations that produce effects similar to oestrogen. However, unlike prescribed drugs, which have their dosage and effectiveness demonstrated in controlled trials, so-called alternative or herbal treatments do not have to undergo this kind of rigorous testing and their effectiveness usually has to be taken on trust or the evidence of anecdote. (Read more about herbal treatment under 'What about non-prescription treatments?' below.) In this book when we use the term 'natural' about hormones we are talking about the kind made by the human body. For more detail on what is in HRT preparations see the box *What's in HRT?* If you are only interested in how they are used and how they work, read on.

HRT comes wearing many different hats

HRT comes in a number of different forms, or formulations, as the drugs industry calls them. If your womb is still in place you need to take both oestradiol (the oestrogen-mimicking hormone) and a progestogen. These hormones are combined in a number of different ways and can enter the body by several different routes: by the mouth, the skin, the vagina or up your nose! It is also possible to have an implant inserted surgically under the skin: this lasts for up to six months. The regime you choose depends partly on the symptoms you experience, partly on your general health, your lifestyle and your temperament. The long-term health implications of taking HRT and the finely balanced decisions each individual has to make on this are covered in Chapter 5. Meanwhile here is a brief summary of the kinds of HRT available.

- *Pills* are probably the most popular way of taking HRT, as not all types are available in other preparations such as a skin patch, a gel or a nasal spray. These usually come in a calendar blister pack that tells you which pill to take each day. Pills are usually the first-choice medication. Your doctor will only move you on to patches or other forms if you have problems with pills.

- *Patches* are clear plastic squares that you stick onto the body somewhere below the waist and above the top of your thigh. Generally speaking, the higher the dose the larger the patch. You change patches once or twice a week on regular days. The drug dose in a patch can be lower than in a pill because it doesn't have to pass through the gut and the liver before getting into the bloodstream. Patches allow oestrogen to be absorbed slowly through the skin providing a more gradual and, in some sense, more natural release than a tablet, although they can occasionally cause skin irritation or an allergic reaction to the adhesive in the patch. There are two sorts of patches: reservoir patches that contain hormones in solution and stick to the skin by an adhesive ring round the edge of the patch, and 'matrix' patches where the hormone is distributed throughout an adhesive layer covering the whole side of the patch. These are slightly less likely to cause skin reactions.

- *Gel* works in the same way as patches; the drug is absorbed via the skin. You rub the gel onto the underside of the upper arms, legs or lower abdomen. It is a bit complicated to use: it must be applied to a different area of the skin each time, allowed to dry and you must not touch the area afterwards for at least an hour, nor apply any other sort of cream or lotion, which could be somewhat limiting if you are in an intimate relationship.

- *Implants* are inserted surgically under local anaesthetic. They release oestradiol over many months and because of this may be inflexible, although they save you having to remember to take a regular dose. This method is more suitable for women who have had a complete hysterectomy because you cannot deliver progestogens via an implant. Women who still have their womb have to take this second, protective hormone by mouth.

- *Nasal sprays*, a relatively recent innovation, have the same limitation. Only oestradiol can be absorbed via this route. You still have to take progestogen pills if you have your womb.

- *Vaginal rings*, impregnated with oestradiol, last for three months at a time. They are inserted into the upper part of the vagina, and can cause discomfort. For women who have had a hysterectomy these single-hormone treatments do have the advantage that they can achieve adequate blood levels with a small dose of the drug.

If you stick to the oral route for taking HRT, you have to decide whether you want to imitate your natural monthly period and have a withdrawal bleed, and if so how often you want it. The oestradiol in the HRT that you take every day has the effect of building up the womb lining. This increases the risk of cancer so you need to take progestogens to protect it. Some regimes recommend that you take progestogens every 10–14 days and then, when you stop, the drop in progestogens signals to the enriched lining of the womb to come away, and you get a withdrawal bleed. You also have the option of taking the course of progestogens once a month, or once every three months – a less familiar pattern, but one that still provides sufficient protection to the lining of the womb – or even less frequently. You can also take the two hormones, oestradiol and progestogen, together, every day, without a break. (A lower dose of progestogen may suffice in this regime.) If you adopt this pattern you may eventually stop bleeding altogether, although some younger women continue to have some spotting for a few months. This formulation is recommended for those who stay on HRT for several years. It is usually offered once an ultra-sound examination has confirmed that the lining of your womb has settled down to being stable and not too thick, what is called *quiescent*.

If you are one of the lucky ones who are not afflicted by any of the tiresome short-term symptoms we have been discussing, you may be aware that even those who don't have symptoms when they go through the change may nevertheless be susceptible to one or other of the increased health risks that affect women *after* the menopause. These permanent changes that take place in the body at this time can lead to long-term health problems like brittle bones. We will look at how HRT affects these conditions and also what other drugs are available to treat specific long-term health risks in Chapters 6–9. These are important if for some reason you are unable to take HRT, or after you stop taking it.

Does anything else work apart from HRT?

Many of the symptoms listed at the beginning of this chapter come down to a failure of the body's heat-regulating mechanism following a fall in oestrogen production. Between 45 and 85 per cent of women experience such symptoms at the menopause. Doctors call them *vasomotor* symptoms, which relates to the fact that a flush is caused by the sudden widening of blood vessels just under the skin. These symptoms are difficult to treat other than with hormones. You can take measures to keep cool, or to cool down when the symptoms strike; avoid tight clothing, stressful situations or having to do things in a rush, but although this may relieve the symptoms it won't cure them. Those who don't suffer from them may be tempted to dismiss hot flushes as nothing more than a physical irritation, such as you feel when you have been exceptionally energetic or find yourself trapped in a hot, enclosed space. However, if left untreated they can lead to a cascade of other more disruptive symptoms: disturbed sleep and exhaustion, leading to irritability and mood fluctuation, anxiety and depression. This has led some experts to speculate that the improved mood many women report after taking HRT is more to do with being able to have a good night's sleep rather than because of the beneficial effects of the hormones per se.

This may explain why mood-altering drugs with sedative side effects like the *selective serotonin reuptake inhibitors* (SSRIs), better known by the trade names Cipramil, Cipralex, Faverin, Lustral, Prozac and Seroxat, are among very few alternatives to hormone treatment for vasomotor symptoms. Studies show that quite low doses of SSRIs can be effective for up to 70 per cent of sufferers. The drug that has been tested most extensively is venlafaxine (Efexor), also an SSRI but with an added effect on another brain *neurotransmitter* (chemical messenger), noradrenaline, although there is also evidence that Prozac works.

Apart from SSRIs, there are drugs based on various forms of progestogen: megestrol (Megace), and medroxyprogesterone acetate (Depo-Provera), that provide some relief from vasomotor symptoms, but both come with drawbacks. The latter has to be given by injection and both can lead to weight gain – the last thing you need when trying to keep healthy after the menopause. There are one or two other drugs that have been used in the past, but they all have side effects out of proportion to the relief they provide. They may not be HRT as currently defined, but they are, of course, still hormones.

What about non-prescription treatments?

All the treatments mentioned so far are available on prescription and manufactured and tested by pharmaceutical companies. But if you read about the menopause either in print or online you will also come across a forest of complementary and herbal cures, widely advertised and recommended. These include several compounds based on plant extracts that act like oestrogen (sometimes called phytoestrogens) and a long list of herbal extracts. Some of these have a strong oestrogen-like effect: motherwort leaf, saw palmetto berry, rhodiola rosea root and red clover blossom are among the most potent, while dong quai root, black and blue cohosh, vitex berry, hops flower, wild yam, and liquorice root have a moderate oestrogen effect. Many of these are sold in health food shops and classified as foods rather than medicines, which means that they don't have to undergo the same rigorous testing regime as prescription medicines before they can be sold. So far only black cohosh and vitamin E have been shown to be effective for vasomotor symptoms, and then only for the short term (six months). While others *may* be effective there is at the moment no evidence of their long-term safety. What is more, because of their oestrogen-like effects they carry the same health risks as drug company oestradiol if you happen to be in one of the high-risk groups.

Painful intercourse

The fall in the production of oestrogen produces changes in the skin and in the *mucus membrane* or *mucosa* – the special skin-like lining of body cavities like the mouth or vagina. Increased levels of oestradiol cue puberty and cause changes in the lining of the vagina to prepare it for intercourse and childbirth, and the fall in production at the menopause leads to the reverse process: the cells lining the vagina get thinner, less elastic and they produce less lubrication, which leads in turn to pain or irritation during intercourse. This physical discomfort can be treated with topical (local) oestrogens in creams (delivered with an applicator like Tampax), or *pessaries* (lozenges that can be placed high in the vagina and dissolve slowly). These preparations raise the levels of hormones locally and improve the condition of the vaginal lining, but do not affect the whole body and are therefore useful for women who are advised not to take systemic (whole body) HRT. Purely mechanical lubrication prior to intercourse can be obtained from vaginal moisturizers like KY jelly or, for that matter, almost any other moisturizing cream.

The medical literature suggests that a lot of women go off sex at the menopause and this is usually attributed to loss of hormones, loss of sensitivity in the vagina and the emotional turmoil that accompanies these changes and that has a knock-on effect on mood, stress, relationships and self-esteem. Some studies suggest that treatment with a low dose of testosterone can help and a large study is currently being conducted in Aberdeen to confirm these findings. But it's as well to remember that sexual desire is related to many things other than hormones. Low libido affects women at all ages, and treating it as a medical condition is only rarely appropriate. If a woman hasn't been enjoying the sex available to her, going through the menopause may seem as good an excuse as any to have less. And for a woman who is enjoying sex there are many things she can do to overcome the problems, apart from taking testosterone, which is associated with quite a few side effects.

Changes in the cells of the vagina also make it less resistant to ulceration and infection and the same changes affect the mucosa lining of the *urethra* – the tube leading to your bladder – causing inflammation and pain when passing water, urgency, frequency, and even stress incontinence (when a small amount of urine escapes involuntarily, for example when you cough or laugh or do something energetic). Loss of oestrogens may also affect the muscles that help hold urine in the bladder (known by the euphemism 'continence' and its opposite 'incontinence'). There is no obvious way to deal with this problem apart from adapting your behaviour and learning not to put things off too long. Difficulty holding back urine is just one of the boring problems you face as you become older. It is not all down to the menopause. More detail on the long-term changes that affect the vagina and the bladder can be found in Chapter 9.

5

Making a personal choice:
is HRT for you?

It is surprisingly difficult to find objective advice about whether to take HRT or not. The problem is that almost everyone – GP, specialist, medical author, website – appears to be in one camp or another: HRT enthusiast or HRT hater. I have to put my hand up and declare an interest here: I really enjoyed taking HRT, had no side effects, and had to be dragged forcibly away from it by a wise GP saying, 'Don't you think, Mrs Pigache, that after 20 years it's time you gave them up?' But I am a single case and am fortunate in having exceptionally good health. What worked for me and for others like me does not delude me into thinking HRT is automatically right for all women.

The medical profession (like my GP) is cautious by nature; not keen to push pills unless they are clearly needed, which means that in all probability the doctors in your life will not push you in the direction of HRT, though they will certainly inform you about it, and very properly emphasize the risks involved. They read the literature and they know that the verdict on who should or should not take hormones for the menopause has swung violently from one pole to another in the past 20 years or so. Your GP will be able to identify whether you are in one of the high-risk groups advised not to take HRT. But only you can analyse your feelings about the experience of the menopause, now and for the rest of your life. Only you can weigh the risks and benefits as they affect you. One woman thinks a few sweaty moments are no big deal, whereas another regards anything that might interfere with her sex-life as anathema. For one woman adding even slightly to the risk of breast cancer is unthinkable, whereas another believes in living for the present, clings to her youth and lets distant risk in the future go hang. And just as everyone can dig up an uncle who has smoked until 90 without dropping dead from lung cancer in order to justify smoking cigarettes, so most women can quote an older friend who has taken HRT until her eighties and appears none the worse, if not better, to support their own choice. I know several.

Read all about it!

Most of us learn about new drugs, and the risks of new drugs, from newspapers or television. These reports are good in that they are couched in simple terms using language that can be understood without having a medical degree or a degree in pharmacology. But they are bad in that they are of necessity brief and simplified and they don't have the space to put new findings into context; nor have their readers the inclination to read that sort of back story. The newspaper stories suffer from another problem: headlines. Headlines have to be even simpler and shorter than a news report in the paper. They are written by sub-editors, who cut and trim the reporter's words so that they fit onto a page, and who do not usually have as much understanding of the science as the writer of the story. Among medical journalists there is a joke that all drug stories go out under one of two headings: 'New miracle wonder drug' or 'Shock, horror, drug probe!' The sub-editor decides if the story is good or bad, and sticks on a dramatic headline that will catch the reader's eye.

It doesn't make for balanced, let alone nuanced reporting. It makes the doctors and scientists who work with drugs spitting mad, and occasionally it leads those people whom the drugs are intended to help make unwise choices based on oversimplified or inaccurate information. This book aims to avoid this sort of oversimplification.

Studying the studies

In Chapter 2 I told you about early experiments using unopposed oestrogens to treat menopausal symptoms. These are now history, but they do demonstrate a trend. The pendulum regarding the use of hormones swings endlessly back and forth and it hasn't stopped yet. Oestrogens based on mare's urine were an amazing advance on ground-up animal ovaries, but further down the line came the 'Shock, horror, probe!' story: they gave women cancer of the lining of the womb. Adding in progestogens appeared to head this problem off at the pass. Not only did women say they felt more youthful, sexy, energetic and positive about life, studies appeared that supported the manufacturer's claim that HRT brought definite health benefits. Once again the treatment's star was in the ascendant.

Early data on health benefits was published in 1985, and came from the Nurses' Health Study – an ongoing study of the health, habits and lifestyle of 120,000 American nurses. It reported on 32,000 of these nurses and included the dramatic discovery that those who were taking HRT were 50 per cent less likely to have had a heart attack than the nurses who were not on it. The finding was confirmed by a follow-up study published in 1991. It reinforced what doctors had always suspected. They knew that up to the age of the menopause women are more than six times *less* likely to have a heart attack than men of the same age. But after the menopause this massive advantage tails off. It made sense that it was the distinctive balance of hormones in a fertile woman's body that conferred this protection, and that therefore taking hormone replacement after the menopause could well prolong the premenopausal advantage.

But there were limitations to the Nurses' Health Study. It was not the kind of trial where one group takes a drug and other takes a dummy pill, a *placebo*, and results are compared: the randomized controlled trial (RCT), which is the gold standard for demonstrating the effectiveness of a drug. (See box, *The gold standard for drug trials*.) It was what is called an 'observational study'; that is, the nurses' habits and health were recorded and assessed scientifically but they made their own choices about what exercise they took, what diet or what drugs or what medical check-ups they had. Because of this, other factors crept in to confound the results. A woman taking HRT was more likely to get regular health checks and to be generally more disciplined about looking after herself. Were the nurses having fewer heart attacks *because* they were on HRT, or were women who were healthier in the first place the ones who chose to take HRT?

The gold standard for drug trials

The idea of using scientific method to test the effectiveness of drugs or other medical procedures is a relatively modern concept. Witch doctors apart, curing people has historically been as much about faith and luck as medical understanding or effective treatment. But as the causes and mechanisms of disease emerged from mystery and superstition, so the physician's ability to alter the course of disease predictably increased: to intervene, to use a favourite medical word.

The first example of what is now regarded as the gold standard for clinical trials, the randomized controlled trial – or to give it its high-carat denomination, the randomized, double-blind, placebo-controlled trial – took place just after World War Two in 1948. Austin Bradford Hill set up a trial of streptomycin, an antibiotic derived from soil fungi discovered a few years previously, to measure its effectiveness in treating TB. Patients with advanced pulmonary (lung) TB were randomly put into one of two treatment groups. Why random? Well, if doctors are allowed to choose which patients receive a new, active drug and which go into the control group on the standard treatment, there will always be a risk that they will put the patients with the best chance of recovery into the active group, thus skewing the outcome. And how 'blind'? If the patients know that they are on a drug they automatically become inclined to feel better, thus also skewing results. But if they are randomly assigned to either the treatment or control group (the group that is *not* treated) they don't know whether they are on the active drug or not, and the trial is known as 'blind'.

If, in addition, the medical team looking after the patient and running the study is not told which patient is in which group, the study is 'double-blind'; neither the patient nor the medical staff know which patient is in which group and therefore cannot demonstrate any hidden psychological bias in favour of the new treatment – or against it. Clinical studies usually measure the effect of a new drug against a *comparator*: either the standard treatment of the day – it would not be ethical to withhold all treatment from a sick person for research purposes – or, in non-fatal conditions (*unlike* TB) they may be measured against a non-active, sugar or dummy pill (a placebo) to conceal from them whether they are taking the active treatments or not. Patients with some illnesses – depression, for example – may show marked improvement when receiving a placebo. This response to treatment, albeit a non-active treatment, is called the placebo effect.

In the Hill study of streptomycin 107 patients were enrolled. When the results were un-blinded it was discovered that 14 of the 52 patients on standard treatment had died (these were very ill people, remember) but that only 4 of the 55 patients who had been given the active drug had died. Streptomycin really worked.

The supremacy of the RCT was reinforced in the early I950s by trials of the Salk polio vaccine tested using an elaborate double-blind trial on nearly two million US children. These early successes, together with early failures of clinical testing procedures – thalidomide, an effective drug for morning sickness in early pregnancy, was found to have damaged the foetus developing in the womb – led to standards for testing experimental drugs being enshrined in European and United States law. These days, before a drug is approved for general use it must be tested against these standards: 'Randomised, placebo-controlled, double-blind trials are the appropriate means, indeed almost the only scientific means, to establish the efficacy of a treatment' (David Healy, *The Antidepressant Era*, Harvard University Press, 1997).

And now for the bad news

And so researchers decided that a rigorous RCT was needed to test the long-term pros and cons of HRT, and particularly to find out whether women on it really were less likely to have heart attacks, when all other things affecting their health were equal. The study was set up by the US National Institutes for Heath and called the Women's Health Initiative or WHI. In 1996 more than 27,340 women were enrolled in the study, the first of its kind. The first part of the study, in which 16,608 women, who still had a womb, took the combined oestrogen/progestogen pill, reported in July 2002 and was an instant sensation. Shock, horror, probe! Yes, there was good news – they had fewer hip fractures and a lower risk of colon cancer – but this was completely eclipsed by the bad news. Not only had more women in the study who had been taking HRT developed breast cancer, they had also had *more* heart attacks and strokes – totally contrary to what was widely expected at the time.

The US health authorities took the unusual step of stopping this part of the study immediately and taking the women in the study off the drug. And, as the news spread, women who had taken HRT convinced it was keeping the worst aspects of middle age at bay were suddenly told to stop.

It caused the most terrible furore in the medical establishment. For 17 years doctors had been telling their patients that although some of the benefits they perceived from taking HRT – more enjoyable sex lives, better skin and hair, prolonged youth even – might be in their mind's eye, the drug would reduce the risk of heart attack and stroke to that of women before they went through the menopause. Some people blamed the drugs companies, others the doctors who had espoused the treatment with too much enthusiasm, and of course some resurrected that old war-horse 'tampering with nature' and castigated women for wanting to fight anno domini. Why couldn't they just grow old gracefully?

But there again ...

But gradually it emerged that perhaps the news was neither as dramatic nor as damning to HRT as had at first appeared. Discerning critics began to point out that the design of the first stage of the WHI had been flawed. And curiously the flaws could be traced to limitations of doing a randomized controlled trial with HRT.

Those designing the trial had faced a number of problems. One key objective was to see the effect of HRT on the incidence of hip fracture, and also on heart attack and stroke – conditions caused by problems with the heart or blood vessels and known collectively as *cardiovascular disease*. Now women go through the menopause between the ages of 45 and 55, and although men might start to drop down from heart attack or stroke at around this age, among women the incidence doesn't start to climb at all until they are well over 55, and they don't face any serious risk until they are over 70. The same goes for hip fracture, the dramatic evidence of osteoporosis – the loss of bone density causing brittle bones – which also does not show up until women are in their seventies. So, if you are doing a trial to test the number of postmenopausal women who have heart attacks and fractures you are going to have to run it for a very long time, and it is going to be extremely expensive.

There was also a problem in using dummy pills (placebos) for the control group in the trial. If you are a woman going through the menopause suffering from beastly symptoms – dripping with sweat at the drop of a hat, thrashing about all night because you can't sleep, bleeding so heavily you dare not leave the house – and you enter a drug trial and are given pills that supposedly will treat these horrible symptoms, and yet they persist, you pretty soon realize you are on the placebo, and in all likelihood you drop out of the trial and go to your GP for the real thing. No, women actually going through the menopause were not suitable subjects for a blind trial; and besides it would not be ethical to keep them from the effective remedy for those symptoms.

And so the researcher decided to enrol older women in the trial: women who were long past the short-term symptoms of the menopause. Older women suffer heart attacks and hip fracture and they don't have menopausal symptoms. The average age of the women in the study was 63, and the majority only started taking the combined drug at least ten years after they had been through the menopause. Only 3,435 were under the age of 55. This meant that it was impossible to separate out risks caused by going through the menopause *without* taking HRT from the risks of taking it rather late in the day. It meant that, in addition, the study took no account of the short-term benefits of HRT during the menopause. And the dose the researcher prescribed for these well-past-the-menopause women was the full dose normally given to women in their late forties or early fifties. (Women who continue to take HRT into their sixties can remain symptom-free on much lower doses of the drugs.)

What the study undoubtedly demonstrated was that it is not, on balance, a good idea to start taking high doses of HRT when you are well past the menopause and on the edge of old age; although there again, it did reduce fractures and the risk of colon cancer. Several other studies had already pointed the way. In 1998 a study called the Heart and Estrogen/Progestin Replacement Study (HERS) – (estrogen is American for oestrogen) – had discovered that HRT was not helpful for women who already had heart disease. Even before the dramatic halt to the first phase of the WHI, the prescribing guidelines for HRT were being updated and doctors were no longer giving it to older women with the goal of protecting them from heart disease. Statisticians have pointed to the fact that the WHI heart data were actually right on the borderline of significance. If you want to read the full story in fascinating detail – and detail is necessary to understand it properly – read Tara Parker Pope's book *HRT: Everything you need to know* (see Further reading at the back of this book.)

Furthermore ...

When the WHI eventually published another part of the trial – that for women on oestrogen alone because they had had their wombs removed – it was found that this drug actually *lowered* the risk of breast cancer by 20 per cent, and what's more these women appeared to experience additional heart protection from using the drug. This good news made fewer waves than the 'Shock, horror, probe' stories. Bad news always makes better headlines than good news.

What these stories illustrate is that we are all individuals, and that some of us are more at risk than others. The best way to approach taking HRT is by drawing up our own personal health profile. This is exactly what a thorough, not too overworked, GP will do.

Drawing up a personal health profile

In calculating risk doctors are aided by tables drawn up with reference to all the major studies of particular health problems. He or she will be helped if you first do some rudimentary calculations of your own, before you consult. Before going into details of the particular health risks that increase after the menopause and looking at how HRT interacts with them, it will help if you take stock of your current health status. Most of us, thank goodness, are not at risk of all the late-life health problems. But there are a number of factors that affect your personal health risks and how you deal with them.

Start with your family history: this gives a clue to where you may be at higher risk. Few diseases are 100 per cent hereditary. Nevertheless, some families have a higher incidence of particular conditions than others, and this seems most likely to be because they share a gene that, in certain circumstances, may make them susceptible to developing a health problem. So if you have blood relations who have had breast cancer, or if several of them have died of heart attack or stroke; or if there is a tendency for older family members to have a hip fracture or to break bones easily, you also may be at risk. Where heart disease is concerned there are a number of classic early warning signs too: do you or members of your family have high blood pressure, high cholesterol, or blood that has a tendency to clot easily?

The next thing, after considering whether you may have any familial high-risk factors, is your current state of health. Do you exercise regularly, are you overweight, are you over-stressed, depressed? Do you (God forbid) smoke cigarettes? Your health now and in the recent past is an indicator of how you may go on. Finally you need to do a psychological inventory. You need to evaluate your priorities in life and your attitude to risk. This is more difficult than you might think. If asked, we would all say that we want to be healthy and are against taking risks with our health, but if you probe deeper you may find that you don't want to be healthy *at all costs*. Would you be prepared to give things up in order to be healthy – for example, flying, drinking wine, making love? Not that you need to give up any of these in order to survive the menopause, but some people clearly do prefer to take risks with their health rather than give something up, otherwise no one would ever smoke cigarettes, get incapacitatingly fat or indulge in binge-drinking. Other people gamble with their savings, take up parachute jumping or just drive too fast and risk an accident or being done for speeding. If you have ever said, 'A short life, but a merry one', you may be among those prepared to take calculated risks. Such things reveal important aspects of your personality that may affect whether you choose to take a drug that may add to your quality of life now, while slightly increasing your risk of certain health problems later.

In each of the next four chapters we will give you a checklist to help you calculate your risk profile and use it to guide you on how you meet those risks. At the end of the book all the risk factors are listed together; you can take this to your doctor for a full discussion should you wish to. It will help you and your GP make well-informed decisions on how you mange the menopause.

6

The menopause and your heart

For 'heart' in the title of this chapter, please read 'heart and blood vessels'. The heart, the blood vessels, the valves connecting those vessels with the heart, and the blood flowing through them, are, for the purposes of this chapter, all part of the 'cardiovascular system'. Diseases of the cardiovascular system are many and varied and some are fatal. (See box, *Know the terms for cardiovascular problems*, for the grisly detail.) The ones that star in the mortality statistics are chiefly heart attack and stroke. Cardiovascular disease is a major killer in Europe and the USA. Although the average woman is unlikely to have a heart attack before her seventies, heart disease or stroke are still responsible for more than half of all female deaths, compared with only one in 25 deaths caused by breast cancer. You need to take care of your heart.

As I have explained, before the menopause women suffer very low rates of cardiovascular disease, but gradually, after the menopause, the incidence increases. This increased risk is partly due to growing older. But another part of it appears to relate specifically to changes in the hormones circulating in the body. It's difficult to be absolutely sure that a woman's distinctive balance of hormones before the menopause is what protects her from heart disease. There are other differences between men and women under 50, though this is the obvious one. But the idea that there is a connection is reinforced by the fact that women whose ovaries are removed in youth, who therefore experience an early menopause, also appear to be at increased risk of heart problems, comparable to much older women. In addition, if women going through a premature menopause and the loss of natural oestrogens take manufactured oestrogens, any increased risk of heart disease disappears. However, the menopause also coincides with other changes in a woman's body not directly attributable to hormones. The first strands of grey in your hair cannot be blamed on oestrogen loss, although it does contribute to a change in hair growth and texture.

Know the terms for cardiovascular problems

We don't expect things to work as well as they get older. Old bangers break down; old boilers have to be replaced, old shoes repaired. Blood vessels have something in common with boilers and motor cars in that they silt up as they age. Fatty deposits, a bit like porridge, begin to build up on the inside of the vessel walls, clogging them and restricting the flow. The deposits are called *atheroma* (Greek for porridge), and the condition is *atherosclerosis*. In addition, the vessel walls begin to lose their elasticity as they age, as do other body tissues like skin. This hardening of the arteries is called *arteriosclerosis*, combining the word 'artery' and 'sclerosis', which is Greek for hardening. As blood negotiates these obstructions it may form clots, and if these clots, or lumps of the fatty deposit break off they can fly to the lungs or the heart causing a heart attack. Or they can fly to the brain causing a stroke.

As the blood vessels become narrower the pressure of the blood flowing through them is increased, causing high blood pressure or *hypertension*. Pushing the blood through narrowed arteries causes all sorts of discomfort and you may suffer from *angina* – pain in the heart. Or because the chambers of the heart have to work harder to pump the blood around narrowed blood vessels they may suffer strain. The fats that are transported around the body in the blood and contribute to the build-up of atheroma are known as lipids – Greek for fat – and one particularly significant form of fat that you will come across is cholesterol.

Fat and cholesterol are carried around combined with protein to make lipoproteins, which, depending on their size and weight, are classified as low-density lipoproteins (LDLs) or high-density lipoproteins (HDLs). It is the LDLs (sometimes called 'bad' cholesterol) that transport cholesterol to body tissue where it can damage arteries. The HDLs are often called 'good' cholesterol. If you have a high level of fats circulating in your blood it's called *hyperlipidaemia* and it puts you at more risk of both atherosclerosis and heart attack. The formation of a clot in a blood vessel is known as a thrombus or *thrombosis*. And finally the tendency of the blood to clot is known as coagulation. This, of course, is not an unhealthy thing when it comes to healing wounds, but it is if clots form in blood vessels.

Both sexes are at increasing risk of cardiovascular disease as they age. A number of factors make you more at risk than others of the same age. Some are part of your basic constitution – for example, your race and certain predispositions you may have inherited from your family. Other factors that affect your level of risk depend on lifestyle choices, like what you eat and drink, whether you take exercise or smoke. The loss of naturally produced oestrogen also almost certainly plays a part in the increased risk among postmenopausal women. Some increased risk may be avoided by taking HRT, some risks may be increased and yet others remain unaffected. It is important to know your risk profile as you approach the menopause and how HRT may or may not affect it. The picture remains complex and confused, as you will by now have realized. And the picture varies between different groups of women.

Hormones and blood lipids

Consider the cardiovascular problems listed in the box *Know the terms for cardiovascular problems*. Middle-aged people of either sex are constantly bombarded with messages about lowering cholesterol. At the menopause pronounced changes occur in the levels of cholesterol circulating in a woman's blood. The HDLs (good) are reduced and LDLs (bad) become greater. LDLs are responsible for the build-up of fatty plaques in the blood vessel walls, thereby narrowing them and putting up blood pressure, gradually hardening them, and in addition increasing the risk that a chunk of plaque or a blood clot may break off and fly to the heart or to the brain. This chain reaction demonstrates how loss of oestrogen can lead to increased risk of heart disease. And, in general terms – I choose my words carefully, and you will see why – taking HRT *can* interrupt this chain of events. However, it does not appear to affect the long-term outcomes. Your risk of heart disease and stroke, in the long term, is not reduced by taking HRT and may even be slightly increased.

A controlled trial carried out in the USA on women aged between 45 and 65, which compared conjugated oestrogens alone (on women who had had a hysterectomy), the combined HRT (which includes progestogens) and a placebo, found that the hormones boosted the good cholesterol and lowered the bad cholesterol circulating in the blood. Adding progestogen slightly damped down the effect of oestrogens alone, but HRT still improved those women's cholesterol profile. (The first step in the chain reaction was corrected.) At the time of the trial (1995) this fitted well with the anticipated health benefits of HRT. So, a follow-up study, carried out with considerably older women (average age 67) who had already been diagnosed with heart disease (a very different group from the one in the first study), looked to see if the benefits of HRT on cholesterol levels were matched by a reduced risk of heart attack. And they were not. In fact, during the first year of taking HRT the women's risk of having a heart attack actually doubled! So one thing was clear, although HRT improved cholesterol levels it didn't reduce heart attacks in *older women who already had heart disease*. It doesn't, however, rule out that HRT (or more precisely, oestrogens) might protect the health of younger women whose hearts are not yet damaged.

We will return to the issue of the timing of when HRT is taken after we have considered other ways the menopause can affect your heart and circulation.

Hormones and blood pressure

Other factors, in addition to the level of cholesterol circulating in the bloodstream, contribute to the increased risk of heart attack and stroke. One of these is raised blood pressure (BP). (See box, *Why is blood pressure so important?*) Ever since it has been possible to measure BP it has been noted that the systolic (higher figure) tends to rise as people get older. During their fertile years women have significantly lower BP than men, but after the menopause it gradually increases until it is roughly the same. How much is this related to oestrogen loss, with its effect upon bad cholesterol levels, and how much is it just part of general ageing? A Belgian study followed a group of 315 healthy women between the ages of 30 and 70, checking their BP regularly, during which time 44 of them went through the menopause. It revealed that there was a small but distinct increase in the systolic BP that could be traced to the menopause itself, though not a change in the diastolic.

Why is blood pressure so important?

You probably know that high BP is a bad thing without knowing exactly what it is. Blood is driven round your body by the beating of your heart. As the oxygenated blood is expelled from your heart the pressure rises to its highest point (the systolic reading); in between beats the pressure falls to its lowest pressure (the diastolic reading). That is why your BP comprises two figures, one higher than the other. If your BP falls too low – if for example you lose a lot of blood – insufficient oxygen may reach the brain and you will lose consciousness. If it runs continually at a higher pressure (rather than going up in response to exercise and effort, when higher pressure is necessary to increase blood flow, and returning to a lower, resting pressure) it puts strain on the blood vessel walls. Over the long term this causes them to grow thicker and harder, and eventually the added effort of pumping blood through this restricted network damages the chambers of the heart so that they become enlarged, damaged and fail.

As you get older some narrowing and hardening of the arteries is inevitable and consequently your BP may rise. In the past it was often said that a normal systolic BP was your age plus 100. But just because it is common does not mean that it is healthy any more than being fatter and more sedentary in later life is healthy. These days it is recognized that even the elderly need to keep their BP within the normal range. At an ideal BP of 120 over 80 (written 120/80) you will be at no increased risk of heart attack and stroke. A reading of 140/90 is considered normal as you grow older and involves a very small increase in the risk of heart attack and stroke, and you may be encouraged to make lifestyle changes, or take medication to reduce it. The higher your BP, the greater your risk. There is still a lot of uncertainty as to why some people have high resting BP. It sometimes goes up when a woman is pregnant. It goes up if we are under stress, but apart from about 5 per cent of high BP which can be traced to kidney disease, it is still a medical mystery. Heredity may play a part, and certainly the narrowing of the arteries in old age. Fortunately there are a number of drugs that can correct it.

However, even though HRT appears to reduce the build-up of the fatty plaques that narrow blood vessels, and keeps them more flexible, it has not been shown conclusively to prevent rises in systolic BP. Some studies have shown a benefit, some none. So, counter-intuitively, no benefit to BP from taking HRT can currently be guaranteed.

Hormones and blood clots

Blood is designed to clot when exposed to the atmosphere so that it will form a scab and stop the bleeding, but if clots form within blood vessels they cause trouble. A blood clot that forms on the blood vessel wall (a thrombus or thrombosis) can break away and block an important artery (a *thromboembolism*). If a clot stops blood getting to your lungs, it is called pulmonary embolism, which can kill you. If it enters the heart it causes a heart attack, or if one goes to the brain, a stroke. Clots are more likely to form if you have atherosclerosis, and also if factors in the blood increase its tendency to clot. There are a number of different clotting factors in the blood and some are favourably affected by taking HRT; however, the overall risk of stroke is not reduced with HRT. It is actually increased, albeit from a *very low rate*. In one study fewer than one woman in every 100 who were taking HRT had a pulmonary embolism over a five-year period (one in every 200 taking a placebo had one in the same study!). Whether women taking only oestrogen have this slightly increased risk has not been demonstrated. Researchers are still looking into it.

There is one other form of blood clot you may have heard of: deep vein thrombosis or DVT. This is the one people worry about when they have to spend a long time sitting in an aircraft at reduced air pressure. The risk of developing DVT is extremely low, at one person in 10,000; nevertheless, on HRT this risk rises to two women in 10,000. The risk is greater for those with a family history of blood clots. A simple blood test can reveal if your blood has a higher than normal tendency to clot and medication can correct it.

Describing very small risk increases

Picturing risk, especially when it is very low, like the risk we are talking about here, is very difficult. It's one of the most difficult things a science writer ever has to explain. We use the number of people likely to suffer – one in 100, one in 1,000 or one in 10,000 – when talking about comparative risk because that gives a clearer picture than using percentages when you are talking about very small numbers and differences. (Two, rather than one, women in 10,000 is a 50 per cent increase in risk – shock, horror, probe!) Remember this when you are considering whether to take one of the increased risks we are discussing with HRT. Compared with getting knocked down outside your own house, they are negligible.

Other factors contributing to cardiovascular disease

Doctors used to think that blocked blood vessels could be blamed entirely on fatty deposits building up on the walls, but recent research has shown that the walls of arteries may become inflamed. The presence of inflammation can be detected by the presence of certain chemicals in the bloodstream. One of them is called *C-reactive protein* (CPR). Another marker for blocked arteries and an indicator that the blood may clot more readily that can be detected in blood is *homocysteine*. Tests for these chemicals will help build up a picture of your risk profile at the menopause.

The risk of stroke is greatly increased if the two major arteries that run up your neck and carry the blood to the brain – the *carotid* arteries – become narrowed. Whereas the narrowing of the arteries that lead to the heart – the *coronary* arteries – can cause pain, narrowing of these important arteries is effectively symptomless. Because they are near the surface the flow through the arteries can be tested to assess the degree of narrowing (*occlusion*), and if necessary it can be cleared surgically.

The beating of the heart is coordinated by low-level electrical impulses. Sometimes the steady rhythm becomes disturbed and one of the chambers of the heart, instead of contracting regularly, quivers ineffectually, which means that the blood pools and may develop clots which can fly to the brain, causing a stroke. This quivering is called fibrillation and the chamber of the heart usually involved is called an atrium (literally an antechamber), so the condition is called *atrial fibrillation*. This is not uncommon as people become older, but it adds to the risk of stroke.

No list of health risk factors is complete without the usual suspects: being overweight, taking insufficient exercise, being under stress and, above all, smoking. A consequence of these major health risks may be *diabetes*, or a condition called metabolic syndrome, which is a blanket term that covers the combined risk factors already alluded to.

When you take HRT is crucial

If your risk profile includes a number of the conditions or behaviours discussed in this chapter it does not mean that you are going to collapse with a heart attack in the near future. Nearly all these conditions – except the hereditary ones – can be treated or altered. And if they are successfully treated, your risk profile returns to normal. What it does mean, however, is that your doctor may not recommend HRT, or may recommend you take it for a short period only, just to see you through the short-term symptoms.

Do you remember the big Women's Health Initiative (WHI) study, which caused all the fuss in 2002 when it demonstrated that contrary to expectation, HRT did not protect women from heart attack and stroke, but might in some circumstances even increase their risk? The first leg of this study, as I explained, looked only at women who had started HRT rather late in the day – at an average age of 63. Since the first phase of the trial, which was suspended, further results have come through and more detailed analyses have been done, and these make much less depressing news. When the women in WHI who had started HRT within ten years of the menopause were looked at as a separate group, it turned out that they actually had an 11 per cent lower risk of heart problems. This is in contrast with the group who started the HRT ten years or more *after* the menopause, who were at a 22 per cent higher risk of heart attack. In fact, if the women who entered the trial when they were *20 years* past the menopause were considered as a separate group, their risk was increased even more, by 71 per cent. The timing of HRT makes all the difference.

The results of the Nurses' Health Study – an observational study, rather than a randomly controlled trial like the WHI – are consistent with this trend. The nurses who took HRT close to the menopause showed reduced risk of heart attack, and those, like the group in the suspended WHI phase who took it long after the menopause, had an increased risk.

These findings suggest that taken close to the menopause, in other words when it is most helpful in dealing with hot flushes, disturbed sleep and painful intercourse, HRT will not increase the risk of heart attack and may even prolong the protection conferred by natural oestrogens. When HRT is taken is absolutely crucial.

On HRT the healthy get healthier, the sick get sicker

Another trend in health risks can be detected in the WHI study, although the numbers of women in these sub-groups was small, which means that the results are not statistically significant. Those in the study with high BP, who were obese or who suffered from diabetes were at increased risk of heart attack, whereas women with a lower body mass index (BMI) – the standard measure of healthy weight – were at a slightly reduced risk. Other studies have also found that women who already have heart disease are also badly affected by HRT. But HRT does not appear to increase the risk of healthy women.

In her book on HRT Tara Parker Pope sums up a much more detailed analysis than I have room for here with this conclusion:

> The healthier you are before you start taking HRT, the healthier you will be while you are on HRT. The risks and the benefit of these drugs seem to be enhanced or worsened depending on the overall health of the woman who uses them. Most important, analyses of data from the WHI and the Nurses Health Study show that the differences in health risk and benefits seen among HRT users disappears when the women follow a healthy diet and get regular exercise. That means that if you are eating well and staying physically active, you simply don't have to worry about how HRT may affect your heart.

Risk factors for having a heart attack*

- Bad lipid/cholesterol profile
- High blood pressure
- Smoking
- Diabetes
- Obesity
- Level of C-reactive protein in blood
- Level of homocysteine in blood
- High stress levels

Risk factors for having a stroke*

- High blood pressure
- Smoking
- Diabetes
- Narrowing of carotid (brain) blood vessels
- Atrial fibrillation
- Obesity

* Figures from the British Menopause Society.

7

The menopause and cancer

Fear of cancer looms large in the popular imagination. Before running through some of the grim statistics that prompt this fear, a word of reassurance: many people who contract cancer actually die from something else. In other words it is not inevitably fatal, and having it diagnosed early makes it all the more likely that you can head it off at the pass with prompt and effective treatment.

Some grim statistics

Cancer is the second most common cause of death in this country, following cardiovascular disease (dealt with in the previous chapter). It is not exclusively a condition that affects older people, nevertheless the cancers that dominate the mortality statistics are those of old or middle age. Among women, breast cancer is the most common cancer, although more women *and* men die from lung cancer, which is less successfully treated. There is a high number of deaths among both sexes from cancer of the lower bowel (known as *colorectal cancer*), although men are more likely to die from cancer of the *prostate* than from bowel cancer.

The number of cases of breast cancer in this country is increasing, but the number of deaths from the disease has declined steadily over the past 20 years. This is possibly a reflection of the greater number of cancers detected early as a result of the NHS breast-screening programme. (See box, *Screening for breast cancer*.) And here is why it becomes so important after the menopause: four out of every five new cases of breast cancer are diagnosed in women over 50, peaking in the 55 to 69 age group. (This also may relate to the breast-screening programme since women under 50, unless they are identified as being particularly at risk, are not currently invited for regular screening.)

Screening for breast cancer

The word 'screening' implies sifting through a large number of people in order to zero in on the few who may have something or be at risk of it. Where cancer of the breast is concerned small patches of abnormal cells may show up that indicate the very earliest signs of cancer, enabling it to be treated before it can get established. Many countries have breast cancer screening programmes because this disease can kill, and detecting it early can prevent this. In the UK, the NHS breast-screening programme provides a free, three-yearly screen for all women aged between 50 and 70. (The goal is to extend this to 47 and 73 by 2012.) Around one and a half million women are screened each year. It is usually carried out locally, in a hospital or mobile unit, and organized by your GP. It involves taking an X-ray of each breast – a mammogram – which is achieved by compressing the breast horizontally between a sort of tray and the X-ray plate that takes the image. It's a bit uncomfortable but not really painful. Small changes in the breast tissue too small to be detected by touch may show up on an X-ray.

Recently screening units have started using digital mammography equipment. This involves recording the image, not on film but on a computer, just as you do with a digital camera. It has several advantages over film X-ray. The technician can make adjustments to the quality of the image while it is being recorded, thereby improving its quality and reducing the need for repeat screening. The digital image is more sensitive, so that it picks up small abnormalities even when the breast tissue is denser, as it is in younger women. Finally the woman having the X-ray is exposed to lower levels of radiation both during a screen and during possible repeat screens.

X-ray breast-screening may also be combined with an ultrasound scan (one where the image is produced by measuring the variable time it takes sound-waves to go through different sorts of tissue and bounce back). Even better, more sensitive results are claimed for mammograms using *magnetic resonance imaging* (MRI), which exploits the fact that different tissues respond differently to a powerful magnet. Extreme sensitivity is particularly important if the scan is carried out to confirm the presence of breast cancer following a routine screening scan.

You might think that there is nothing to be said against screening, but there are some experts who argue that a screening programme of all woman of a certain age risks picking up growths so small that they are not potentially harmful, leading to a woman being subjected to unnecessary treatment – some of it quite unpleasant. This view is based on the fact that many women who have died of something quite different have been found to have small, non-invasive growths in their breasts that caused them no trouble while they were alive. It's obviously a risk, and one you should be aware of. Whether that leads you to ignore breast screening will more reasonably depend on whether you discover that you are one of those likely to be at risk of the disease.

Risk factors for breast cancer

Understanding the causes of cancer is probably the major medical challenge of our age. There are many different sorts of cancer, and many different causes or combination of causes of cancer. The reason the disease preoccupies scientists now rather than 150 years ago is that in the developed countries we are all living longer, and cancer, like the other big killer diseases of our time, is more common as we grow older. Age is, in fact, the primary risk factor for breast cancer. Ethnic origin may also play a part. In the UK, women whose families came from South Asia have a lower risk of breast cancer than the rest of the population, although this could be due to life-style factors, such as a vegetarian diet and low alcohol consumption. In common with other forms of cancer, the risk factors for breast cancer are partly constitutional – does it run in your family, is there a genetic trait that makes you more vulnerable than average – and partly behavioural – what things have happened in your life that may expose that vulnerability? Great progress has been made in my lifetime in identifying breast cancer genes, but even before this it was recognized that the disease ran in families and a genetic link was suspected.

If you have female relatives who have suffered from cancer your GP may suggest that you are tested for the known breast cancer genes long before you reach the menopause, because although the disease is more common among women after the menopause some 8,000 women (just under 18 per cent of the total) get it when they are younger. However, the vast majority – 95 per cent – of breast cancers have no hereditary cause. The older you or your relatives are when diagnosed, the less likely it is that an inherited gene is the direct cause. You can find out about breast cancer genes at the CancerHelp UK website (the link is provided at the end of this book). A brief outline is provided in the box *Breast cancer genes*.

Breast cancer genes

There are several gene faults that may increase your risk of getting breast cancer above women in the general population. Women with a strong family history of the disease can be tested for the presence of several known faulty genes. (These are variations or mutations of genes that everyone has.) BRCA1 and BRCA2 are gene mutations responsible for somewhere between 30 and 50 per cent of hereditary breast cancer. About half of those carrying these mutations will go on to develop breast cancer by the time they are 50 years old. You can be tested for two other faulty genes – the TP53 gene and the PTEN gene – which are much rarer than the BRCA mutations but also increase the risk of developing breast cancer. There are a few other gene variations that increase the risk of breast cancer by a very small amount.

There is little you can do if you have a genetic predisposition to breast cancer except be alert and have regular scans to detect the early warning signs. Some of the other things that put you at risk are also if not beyond your control then at least very difficult to control. They relate mostly to your reproductive history. If you start your periods early and/or go through the menopause late (they usually go together), you are at increased risk. If you have no children, few children; children late in your life and children you don't breastfeed, you are also more at risk. Then there are things you do have some control over. If you have used oral contraceptives, are using HRT, you slightly increase your risk, as is the case if you are obese, drink too much alcohol or smoke the dreaded cigarettes. (See box, *Factors that increase the risk of breast cancer*.)

Factors that increase the risk of breast cancer

Factors are listed in order of significance.

- Menopause occurred after you were 55 (doubles your risk from average).
- No children before the age of 30.
- Obesity following the menopause.
- Periods started before the age of 11.
- Drink more than three units of alcohol each day.
- Combined HRT for more than five years.

None of these factors increases your risk of breast cancer as much as the familial, gene-related factors. The National Institute for Health and Clinical Excellence (NICE) has attempted to quantify the additional risk of developing breast cancer. It divides women into three groups. All women are at *some* risk of developing breast cancer merely because they have breasts – some men even develop it, though not many – but they are at a *low* risk. (If you like putting numbers to this, one woman in every nine is likely to develop breast cancer at some time in their life.) You are classed as being at a *moderate* risk of developing cancer (in numerical terms that is one women in every six) if the following applies to you.

- A mother *or* sister is diagnosed with breast cancer before the age of 40.
- A mother *or* sister and a more distant relative, but from the same side of the family, are diagnosed with it after the age of 50.
- Two close (mother/sister) relatives are diagnosed after the age of 50.

You get the idea: the quantity and the closeness of relatives affected by the disease and their being on the same side of the family all add up to a gradual increase in the risk of you getting it. It isn't higher maths. The same principle applies to the way NICE classifies those of a *more than moderate* risk of developing breast cancer – in this group two women in every six is likely to develop the disease.

- Two close (mother/sister) relatives are diagnosed before average age of 50.

- One close, plus one more distant relative, average age 50, are diagnosed.
- Three or more relatives of any kind are diagnosed at any age.

A link for NICE breast cancer guidelines (a bit complicated) can be found with further information at the end of this book.

If there is breast cancer in your family there's no need to panic. These are only guidelines, and following an expert assessment by a specialist breast clinic many women turn out to be no more at risk of breast cancer than average. But it does mean that if there is breast cancer in your family you should be assessed, and it also obviously affects whether you decide to take HRT, and for how long, when you hit the menopause. If you are diagnosed as being in an at-risk group you will probably start having yearly mammograms at the age of 40, well before you go through the menopause. If you are identified as being at risk earlier than 40 you may be recommended to have an MRI scan because this technique is better at detecting the early changes in the breast that precede cancer, when the breast is denser, as it is in younger women.

Hormones and breast cancer

Without going into technical detail, it is worth considering why the female breast is so vulnerable, even on average, to cancer. One explanation probably lies in the fact that part of its normal function involves cyclical changes in the tissue of the breast. The middle tissue of the fertile woman's breast is constantly being put on stand-by for the production of a baby and ultimately the production of milk, and then being told to stand easy because the reproduction is off. This switching on and off of changes in the breast, master-minded of course by hormones, opens the door to the possibility of the wrong sort of cells reproducing themselves. There are indications that in a primitive situation, where a woman was more or less pregnant and lactating most of her fertile life, the breasts accommodated the cycle more successfully. Certainly the more children you have and the longer you breastfeed them the lower your chance of breast cancer – other things being equal.

The oral contraceptive and hormone replacement drugs use chemicals that mimic the hormones produced naturally by the woman's body and their prolonged use appears to increase the risk of breast cancer, not to mention blood clots and stroke. Stronger doses of hormones are required to prevent pregnancy and, in addition, a fertile woman may potentially use an oral contraceptive for the best part of her reproductive life. She is, however, younger and hence less vulnerable to cancer than a woman taking HRT after the menopause. Women who started using oral contraceptives before the age of 20 have been shown to have a slightly higher risk of cancer. Where HRT is concerned the studies also suggest that taking it for longer – hence to a greater age, and we can't be sure which is more significant – is riskier. Here's what we know at the moment.

All other factors (that is, familial risk) being equal, taking combined HRT carries the following risks.

- It slightly increases your risk of breast cancer, above the low 17 women in 100 baseline.
- The risk is slightly greater for women over 60.
- The risk increases over time: less than five years increases it very little; up to ten years a little more; over ten years (when you become over 60) more noticeably.
- Five years after you stop HRT your risk is the same as someone (of the same age) who has never taken it.
- If you take the oestrogen-only pill the jury is still out; some studies find a very slightly increased risk, some none at all.

You see where this is leading? Most doctors will support the use of HRT for five years following the menopause, while you are at a low risk of breast cancer, not to mention heart disease, but at a very high risk of nasty temporary conditions like hot flushes, painful intercourse and disturbed sleep. You may also find a GP prepared to give it to you for another five years if your general health is good. After the age of 60 most GPs will ask you to stop. It will have seen you through the tough times by then.

Other cancers after the menopause

As we have explained, cancer is predominantly a disease of the elderly. In England fewer than 1 per cent of cases occur in children and only a quarter in people under 60. The menopause and/or HRT, as distinct from old age, are a factor in only a few cases.

Colorectal cancer – that is, of the lower parts of the digestive tract: the colon and the rectum – is the third most common cancer among women after breast and lung cancer. In this country five or six women in every 100 have a chance of developing it. (Twice that number are at risk of developing breast cancer.) In the USA colorectal cancer accounts for 10 per cent of all cancer deaths among women each year, compared with about 15 per cent due to breast cancer. Your chance of contracting the disease leaps when you turn 50. The mighty noise over the slightly increased risk of breast cancer among those taking HRT has tended to overshadow the good news that the treatment offers distinct protection against colorectal cancer. It's almost 50 per cent lower among those taking HRT than among those who have never taken it. There is a similar link between those who have taken oral contraceptives, which contain similar and even stronger versions of the hormones in HRT, and a lowered risk of developing colorectal cancer. The WHI study found a 44 per cent lower risk for those on the combined HRT pill, but they did not find any difference between those not taking hormone replacement and those on oestrogen alone (women who had had a hysterectomy). This may be because so many women came off the treatment early in the study. Scientists are not sure why HRT should protect against the disease. One theory is that the hormones may lower the concentrations of bile in the bowel. Bile plays an important role in breaking down fat in the gut but it is a powerful irritant to the gut lining.

We explained that it was discovered that taking oestrogen alone greatly increased the risk of getting cancer of the lining of the womb – the endometrium. These days women are only prescribed unopposed oestrogen as a treatment for the menopause if they no longer have a womb. Oestrogen encourages the build-up of the cells that line the womb and this increases the risk of cancer. However, the inclusion of progestogen in HRT greatly reduces this risk. Women who take progestogens for fewer than ten days each month reduce their risk, but only slightly. By contrast those who take it for more than ten days a month experience no increased risk of the cancer at all. This was confirmed by the WHI study. Women often start with the alternating cycle of HRT, which involves a monthly withdrawal bleed, but convert to continuous low-dose progestogens once the endometrium has become stable and not too thick – what is called quiescent.

The relationship between hormones and cancer of the ovaries is rather confusing. Women who take oral contraceptives are told that they actually protect against ovarian cancer. This is because the contraceptive stops them ovulating, and it is the monthly build-up and destruction of cells in the ovaries that can trigger the development of the wrong, harmful cells – a sort of cancerous mistake. However, once you go through the menopause you have stopped ovulating. Early observational studies, and the more recent randomly controlled trials like WHI, do not agree. The problem is that ovarian cancer, unlike cancer of the breast or lower bowel, is rare, so that studies even of large numbers of women do not see a sufficiently large number of cases to make significant comparisons. A recent ongoing study in this country called the Million Women study did find a slightly increased risk among HRT users compared to those who were not taking it, and especially among those taking it for longer periods. It showed that for every 2,500 women taking HRT one more might get ovarian cancer than among 2,500 women not taking it.

Ovarian cancer is rare, but it is difficult to detect and can kill just because it is often detected so late. Probably only those who have a family history of the disease have reason to fear an increased risk from taking HRT to see them over the short-term symptoms of the menopause.

Cancer of the womb, as opposed to cancer of the lining of the womb, is even rarer, and faces the same problem in research studies: there are so few cases it is difficult to make a clear judgement as to how taking HRT affects its occurrence. By and large, however, this seems to be one of the cancers that are actually reduced by HRT.

8

The menopause and your bones

You are by now familiar with me reminding you repeatedly that, because the menopause coincides with the gradual process of ageing, it is difficult to separate the changes directly attributable to the event itself from those that would occur even if your hormones were miraculously to continue in the same pattern as they had for the previous 40 years. Ageing follows maturity as night follows day. One part of a woman's reproductive ageing starts before she is born! A female *foetus* has 6 to 7 million eggs at the 20-week development stage. At the time of birth that number has been reduced to 1 to 2 million, and by puberty, when they might actually get the chance to get fertilized, only 400,000 viable eggs remain. This process of attrition continues during the fertile years, and by age 30 the monthly hormonal cycle that releases eggs and clears the womb lining also begins to run down gradually.

And so it is with the condition of your bones. Bones, like skin and many other organs in the body, are maintained by a process of cell replacement: new cells are produced and old cells reabsorbed. (See box, *Bone building, bone reabsorption.*) The body builds bone rapidly during infancy, slows down a little during childhood and then picks up again in adolescence (the 'growth spurt'). This is why it is so important for children to have a diet rich in calcium, the bone-building element in food. Most bone-building activity is complete by the age of 18, although some modulation and fine-tuning continues for the next decade. Hormones like oestrogen and testosterone contribute to the building boom in youth and play an important part in cell replacement. Somewhere around the age of 30 this relay race of cell turnover slows down. At this age your bones have reached a peak mass – they are at their most strong and dense, but gradually demolition overtakes reconstruction, and little by little bone becomes less dense, lighter and more at risk of breaking. If the loss of density is extreme it becomes the condition known as osteoporosis – or porous bones.

Bone building, bone reabsorption

In some ways the body is like a river: it looks more or less the same over time, but the material it is composed of – water in the case of a river, cells in the case of a human being – is constantly changing. With a few exceptions, the cells that make up the various organs of the body replace one another continuously in a kind of relay race throughout life: they mature, they grow old, they die, and new ones take their place. In bone, cell scavengers called *osteoclasts* break down and remove old bone. When they have done their job they either die or move on to another location. Meanwhile the bone that has become exposed attracts other bone cells called *osteoblasts* which lay down new bone. Normally the amount of bone laid down matches perfectly the amount that is removed. But if the osteoclasts go into overdrive or if the osteoblasts work to rule, then bone loss occurs. This happens in some inflammatory joint illnesses like rheumatoid arthritis, and also in osteoporosis. Healthy bones have a thick outer shell and a strong inner mesh-like structure filled with a connective tissue called collagen, calcium salts, other minerals, blood vessels and bone marrow. In osteoporosis the holes in the bone mesh become bigger, making it more vulnerable to breakage.

The whole skeleton can be affected by osteoporosis, but the fractures that occur most frequently or cause most problems are to the wrist, the spine and the hip, and affect predominantly women over 60. Osteoporosis is more than six times as common among women as among men. Estimates suggest that up to 50 per cent of women fracture a bone at some time after the menopause.

Oestrogens and bone

And once again it can be blamed on oestrogen – or the lack of it. Bone loss in women may start as early as the forties. (A drop in the production of oestrogen may also occur from this age.) At the menopause, however, it accelerates by a factor of ten over the following ten years. On average, women have lighter bones than men to start with. (Size is a factor in your susceptibility to the condition.) They are also slightly less likely to have engaged in the sort of load-bearing or athletic activity that tends to boost bone mass during adulthood. Nevertheless, most of the general vulnerability of the sex in old age can be put down to the fall in the production of oestrogen (oestradiol, to be precise). Part of the evidence for this is that it occurs earlier among women who have had a hysterectomy, and that replacing the oestrogen with HRT following the menopause, at any age, prevents bone loss quite dramatically.

How oestrogen affects the regulation of bone loss or bone building is still something of a mystery. Oestrogen modulates the interactions between the osteoclasts and the osteoblasts. Following the menopause they get out of sync. Tara Parker Pope employs a useful metaphor, saying that oestrogen (and in this case you can take oestrogen to mean not just the natural stuff but the conjugated oestrogens that are part of HRT) is 'essentially the construction site foreman, telling the osteoblast workers to get moving and start building bone'. At the last count, whether oestrogen acts upon the osteoblasts, kicking them into action, or on the osteoclasts, by holding them back, it is clearly a Good Thing for Bones.

What are the symptoms of loss of bone density?

From the point of view of the doctors, the primary symptom is that more old ladies break their wrists, or their spine or hips, thereby landing up in hospital and possibly developing even more serious problems, than old men or younger women. But you don't need to wait until this has happened to discover if you are at risk. One symptom of weakened bone, short of an actual break, can be a fine hairline fracture of the wrist or ankle, which develops in response to stress and in the absence of the more obvious trauma needed to cause a break. This sort of crack may not show up on a regular X-ray, even though the joint will become swollen and painful.

For many women, loss of bone density does not constitute a health hazard. During a healthy, active adult life you can build up a fairly comfortable cushion of bone density that will allow for some loss in old age. If after the menopause you continue being active and eating well, avoiding the dreaded cigarettes, you may go to your grave with all bones intact. The definition of osteoporosis has changed slightly over the years. In the past you were not considered to have it unless you had suffered a fracture that could be attributed to bone loss. These days we have bone-density screening and the bones of a woman in her fifties may be compared with those in their twenties, thirties and forties, and yes, even if unbroken, they are less dense. In addition we have a drugs industry keen to supply treatments for widespread conditions, which means that women, and more particularly doctors, are subjected to drug marketing overkill. This inevitably affects attitudes to risk, and to treatment.

Who is at risk?

After the reassurance come the warnings. Some women are more at risk of osteoporosis than others. These are some of the risk factors you should know about.

- *Have you had an early menopause?* Whether you go through the menopause naturally before the age of 45, or because of a hysterectomy, the result is a loss of oestrogens and your risk of osteoporosis is increased.
- *Does a female relative have osteoporosis?* Genes play their part in many medical conditions. They make you more susceptible to a condition even though you may be able to avoid becoming a victim by modifying your behaviour. Your genes almost certainly contribute to the age at which you go through the menopause and whether you have a delicate bone structure. If your mother had a hip fracture before the age of 80 there is a high risk that you will develop osteoporosis too.
- *Are you thin or tall?* Although the disadvantages of being over-weight overshadow the advantages, not being too thin, or *not losing* weight, has also much to recommend it in later life. Older women who weigh less than they did at 25 are twice as likely to suffer a hip fracture as the average woman. Interestingly, height also plays a role. Perhaps because you have further to fall; perhaps because managing long limbs becomes more difficult as you age.
- *What do you eat and drink?* Calcium and vitamin D are essential for normal bone growth and deficiencies in these can lead to

osteoporosis. In this country, and even more so in Scotland, we can be cruelly deprived of sunlight – the principal source of vitamin D. Although sunburn can raise the risk of skin cancer, a shortage of vitamin D is increasingly being found to be associated with a whole range of other illnesses. If you drink too much caffeine (in coffee, tea and cola) you may also increase your risk of osteoporosis. Caffeine leaches calcium from bones. But don't think that knocking the booze is any better; heavy indulgence in alcohol is known to inhibit bone-building osteoblasts.

- *Are you taking enough exercise?* Women who walk regularly have been found to be at 30 per cent lower risk of hip fracture than those who don't. Physical activity increases bone strength. If you can't get out of a chair without using your hands, be warned. On the other hand, it appears that if you spend more than four hours a day on your feet, just standing, you are at increased risk compared with those who walk.
- *Do you smoke?* Health writers get tired of saying it: smoking damages your health and in this context it also impairs bone growth.
- *Have you been ill or had to take certain medication?* Being ill often reduces bone density. Being confined to bed for a long time certainly affects it. In addition, some drugs, like the *corticosteroids* (the anti-inflammatory kind of steroid, not the anabolic kind used by weight-lifters) which are prescribed as long-term treatment for conditions such as asthma, rheumatoid arthritis or ulcerative colitis, put you at a high risk of developing osteoporosis.
- *Is your bone density low?* In Chapter 3 we discussed the tests you may undergo at the menopause. If you are found to have a high-risk profile for osteoporosis your GP will probably suggest you have a bone-density scan. Women in one US study who had low bone density on a scan were found to be 60 per cent more at risk of hip fracture. However, women who had *no other* risk factors, apart from a low bone-density scan, had only a 2.6 per cent increased risk.

It is important to recognize that low bone density, as demonstrated on a scan, is just a single risk factor. It is a combination of several risk factors that makes you notably at greater at risk of hip fracture. In the US study 66 per cent of the fractures recorded happened to women with more than one risk factor.

Treating bone loss

It is because of its demonstrable role in avoiding osteoporosis that HRT managed to stay in the doctors' good books. When it was greeted as a 'youth elixir' this advantage was not at first noted, but the Women's Health Initiative (WHI) – the same study that took women off the treatment early because it appeared that it was not reducing their risk of heart attack and stroke but actually increasing it slightly – was the first to demonstrate that oestrogen drugs not only improved bone density but that this translated into a lower risk of broken bones. The women on HRT in this study (remember they were mostly older women, and therefore at more risk of broken bones) had a 33 per cent lower risk of hip fracture. Those on oestrogen alone had a 35 per cent lower risk. The reduction of risk was most pronounced among thinner women (those with a body mass index below 25), a group more at risk to begin with. Those women who also took a calcium supplement every day (1,200 milligrams) reduced their risk still further. The advantage of taking HRT was more dramatic for those at a high risk of bone fracture than for those at lower risk. The researchers calculated that for women at a high risk of bone fracture the benefit of taking HRT outvoted the slightly increased risk of stroke or heart attack and the increased risk of breast cancer. For those at a lower risk of broken bones the choice was not as clear.

Unfortunately the research also showed that the protection conferred by HRT wore off after women came off it. Five years later their risk profile had returned to what it was before they took it. So, just when the drug firms thought that a major USP was within their grasp, they had it snatched away again. But they didn't give up. Much study then (about ten years ago) went into a hunt for a low-dose version of hormone replacement that would protect the bones of vulnerable women without increasing their risk of other health problems. A low-dose oestrogen patch (10 microgram – that's half the dose of most oestrogen-patch drugs), marketed under the name Menostar, was tested. A two-year study, funded by the drug manufacturer, found that bone density had been increased by about 3 per cent in women's spines and by about 1 per cent in their hips. The study did not go on long enough to see if this translated into a lower rate of actual bone fracture as it had in the WHI research.

It follows, therefore, that even if you do take HRT – and we return to making this difficult decision later – if you have more than one risk factor for osteoporosis you really need to find an acceptable long-term treatment. Consider first the lifestyle adaptations discussed in broader terms in Chapter 10. Regular, weight-bearing exercise – walking, DIY, gardening, taking the stairs not the lift – will help you build bone, and muscle to support your joints. It will also help you maintain a steady weight: not too heavy but not too thin either. Some supplements have also been shown to help. Calcium (an average of 1,500 mg per day is recommended after the age of 60) and vitamin D, usually recommended at 400–800 international units (IU) a day to begin with, will reduce the risks of fracture of the hip, wrist and spine. The vitamin D helps bones absorb calcium. Consuming calcium alone is not enough; you have to make sure it gets into the bone if it is to boost strength. Latterly some experts have recommended that during the winter months, when you are unlikely to get enough natural sunlight to boost your own production of vitamin D, 1,000 IU a day, or even more, may be desirable. These are all things you can do without recourse to a doctor.

Other drugs that reduce bone loss

If your osteoporosis risk profile calls for it, your GP may recommend various forms of prescription medication. First line of defence is usually a group of drugs called *bisphosphonates*, of which the most common is alendronic acid, although there are other versions. These act by inhibiting osteoclast activity, thus slowing the breakdown of bones. Alendronic acid is not everyone's cup of tea. Some people find it difficult to swallow and there are a number of contraindications (situations that rule out taking it): for example, if you have kidney problems or have suffered from a stomach ulcer or other digestive problems. Side effects include heartburn, diarrhoea, constipation and abdominal discomfort. If it is prescribed for you, follow the instructions for taking it carefully, but if you really can't stomach it, ask your doctor for an alternative.

There is another group of drugs called *selective oestrogen receptor modulators* (SERM – the US spelling of oestrogen drops the initial 'o'), of which the best known is raloxifene. This is not a hormone treatment but it mimics the actions of oestrogen, and in a selective way: it acts beneficially upon bones, but at the same time blocks the effects of oestrogen on either the womb, stimulating the cells of the endometrial lining, or the breasts. This lowers the risk of endometrial and breast cancer associated with HRT. Another SERM, raloxifene's close relative tamoxifen, is the first-line treatment for breast cancer. Side effects are very much those of the menopause itself, because it selectively blocks some oestrogen receptors: hot flushes, vaginal discomfort, leg cramps, constipation and difficulty in controlling the bladder upon exertion. You definitely don't want to be taking a SERM while actually going through the menopause. But fortunately bone fracture only becomes a problem for women at a much later age – over 60, or even later.

The latest drug aimed at reducing bone loss is strontium ranelate, a dual action bone agent. Unlike the bisphosphonates, which act by inhibiting osteoclasts, strontium ranelate stimulates osteoblast activity in addition to inhibiting osteoclasts. This dual action – bone building as well as damping down bone loss – more closely resembles the natural process of bone-cell turnover that operates during adult life. Five-year studies of this drug suggest that it not only reduces bone loss but reduces the incidence of fracture for all age groups. The only people advised not to take it are those who have suffered or are at clear risk of a vein thrombosis. Familiar side effects – nausea, diarrhoea, eczema and headaches – affect very few people and tend to disappear after three months. At the moment this drug is only approved in England for the treatment of at-risk women who cannot tolerate alendronic acid.

What treatment should I choose?

The decision about how to treat the menopause is overwhelmingly an individual one. It depends on your individual health, your risk profile, your lifestyle, your attitude to risk, and, once you actually have treatment, your response to the drug.

Making such decisions is extremely complex and I hope to pull all the threads together at the end of the book (see Chapter 10, 'At the menopause: the HRT decision' in particular). But to some extent what you do about preventing bone loss is simpler than some other decisions. Risk profile apart, every woman going through the menopause should be taking stock of her lifestyle – eating a balanced diet, taking plenty of exercise, maintaining a steady weight, moderating the booze and (if she hadn't already done it) giving up cigarettes. If the short-term symptoms hit you badly, and your health profile doesn't completely rule it out, we suggest that you try HRT for a few years, to get you over the worst of it. If you are able to take HRT, that takes care of the problem of bone loss *while you take it.* When you stop taking it some alternative form of protection may be required, and then only if you have several risk factors. Take guidance from your GP. Supplement with calcium and vitamin D first; then try alendronic acid if it is recommended, and only move on to one of the other (more expensive) drugs if you cannot tolerate it – but do let the doctors know if you really can't.

9

Meanwhile, in another part of the body

As I warned you, hormones operate just about everywhere. Most obviously they control your menstrual cycle, but also, as we have explained, they affect blood vessels, fats circulating in the bloodstream, bones, breasts, brain and many more things that impact powerfully upon your health and well-being. When oestrogen production drops, a raft of body processes change in its wake. In this chapter we round up some health problems in other parts of the body.

Hormones and the vagina

Oestrogen plays an important part in maintaining the strength, elasticity and plumpness of both external skin and the mucous membrane – the lining of body cavities. The most widely reported symptom of falling oestrogen production upon these organs is discomfort during intercourse. Fortunately not everyone experiences this problem. (More about who does below.) Discomfort during intercourse is not exactly illness, of course, so it tends not to attract much attention from doctors compared with serious health hazards like fractured hips or heart disease. However, at the University of Melbourne in Australia they have done a number of studies of both physical discomfort and the broader picture of sexual satisfaction during and after the menopause. They discovered that whereas only 3 per cent of women have a problem with vaginal dryness during their fertile years, by the onset of the menopause the number jumps to 21 per cent, and by the time they are past the menopause it becomes 47 per cent – nearly half of all women questioned! This does not make the front page in most accounts of menopausal problems. Nor does a handicapped sex life rate as a priority for most overworked doctors, though in my opinion it is important at any time, and particularly at this time of life. There are many factors that contribute to a satisfactory sex life. Here and now we deal with changes to the mucosa and its role in physical discomfort. In Chapter 10 we will look at other, vital components in your sex life, like an arousing partner and enjoyable love-making. The vagina and adjacent areas are not a woman's only erogenous zones – areas where sexual excitement is registered. The brain is just as important, and hormones are at work there as well.

A fall in the production of oestrogen (oestradiol) causes other changes that affect the vagina in addition to reduced lubrication. There is reduced blood flow to the vaginal wall (increased blood supply is a natural response to arousal), a weakening of the muscle wall and a thinning of its lining. All parts of the genital organs become thinner and smaller after the menopause. The thinning, combined with a loss of elasticity, can make the mucosa prone to irritation, soreness or, if you don't find a substitute source of lubrication, actual damage. Similar changes affect the urinary tract and the bladder – they become smaller and the membrane lining them thinner, a process called atrophy (a loss of size or strength). There is also a subtle alteration in the balance of chemicals in both vagina and urinary tract, leading to an increased risk of infection, and of leakage from the bladder.

It sounds depressing but hopefully you won't notice the difference because it happens gradually over some years. HRT successfully defers changes to the mucosa and the attendant problems, while you take it. It's not the only treatment, but it is the only treatment to hit a number of problem-birds with the same stone, so to speak. Scrupulous attention to personal hygiene will reduce the increased risk of infections and effective substitutes for lubrication are available. You don't have to use the less than aesthetic KY jelly; I have friends who tell me that the smell of Nivea, or whatever cream they go for, becomes quite a turn-on, and there is a proprietary product – a bioadhesive moisturizer – called Replens that actually rehydrates the tissues. (They don't say if it works on the face.) You will, however, ultimately have to get used to peeing more often.

The experts of the University of Melbourne Women's Midlife Health Project, who carried out much of the research into women's sexual health at the menopause, say that reduced lubrication may even have an upside, since the problem can be solved by taking longer over foreplay, which improves sexual relationships. They say that for some women sex after the menopause becomes wonderfully stress-free. Anxieties about pregnancy, periods, not to mention the distraction of young children, become a thing of the past.

It is very important to keep up a healthy sex life at this age. Just as muscles can waste away if you lie in bed, unable to use them, so it goes with the vagina. Use it or lose it, as the saying goes. Women who are more sexually active suffer less vaginal atrophy, plus all the consequent discomfort and health problems. One study compared postmenopausal women who were having sex three or more times a month with those having it fewer than ten times a year. The sexually active women had healthier, younger vaginas than their sexually abstinent sisters.

Hormones and the skin

There does not unfortunately seem to be any reliable way of exercising the skin on your face or hands in order to preserve it. Oestrogen depletion has the same effect on the skin as on the mucosa, though if your vagina gets thin, bloodless and dry at least you can't see it. Skin becomes thinner, drier and less resilient; the plump padding just below the surface loses its bounce and elasticity, making the skin above more prone to wrinkles. It's a gradual process starting for some women before the menopause, but afterwards the need to protect and moisturize the skin becomes even more important. Not being strictly speaking a health problem, and certainly not a life-threatening one, the effect of the menopause on the skin has also not received a great deal of medical attention, and women are for the most part too shy to ask their doctors about it. You will hear plenty of anecdotal evidence for the fact that the skin deteriorates after the menopause and that HRT preserves it, but few studies have investigated it. The old problem arises: is it the loss of oestrogen per se that causes changes to the skin, or is it anno domini? (See box, *A few facts about skin*.)

A few facts about skin

This skin is the body's largest organ. It measures as much as two square metres on an adult man and about one and a half square metres on the average woman. It's about 70 per cent water – which explains why moisture retention is important to keep it in good condition. It comprises three layers: the outer layer is known as the *epidermis* (from the Greek for 'outer' and 'skin'). The cells in the epidermis are completely renewed every month. New cells, formed beneath the skin, gradually progress through the layers until they appear in the epidermis, finally to be sloughed off as dead skin cells, or follicles. New cells also form to heal any damage to the skin. The middle layer of the skin is the dermis, a dense, flexible layer of connective tissue cells and collagen fibres. Collagen is found throughout the body and performs a variety of functions, but 'padding' is one of its principal roles. It is collagen that gives skin its firmness and resilience in youth but loses elasticity as you age. As well as collagen the cells of the dermis contain substances called elastin and *hyaluronic acid* (HA), the water-retaining element in skin. The nerves that provide your sense of touch are also located in the dermis. Beneath the dermis is the deepest layer of the skin, the *subcutis* (under-skin): a thick cushion of connective tissue held together by collagen fibres that contains fat cells and blood vessels and acts as an energy reservoir, protective padding and heat insulation all rolled into one. This layer also connects the skin to the various underlying tissues of the body.

Hair grows in skin – both the hair and the nails, which are made from the same protein, keratin, are also affected by oestrogen loss after the menopause. The most obvious change to your hair is the gradual loss of colour, but hair growth also slows down, hair becomes thinner and the texture changes in response to depleted oestrogen. HRT will usually delay these effects, but hair loss can be caused by other things like a malfunctioning thyroid gland, which often affects women at this time, stress and various sorts of medication.

People and faces do not all age at the same rate or in the same way, and this becomes more noticeable the older they get. It's easy to tell the age of a child, slightly more difficult when children become adolescents. More difficult still in their twenties and increasingly so through the decades until, by 65, even an experienced health practitioner finds it near impossible to calculate exactly someone's chronological age compared with their physiological age – which may be greater or less depending on a number of factors. Genes and life behaviour obviously play a part. When did your mum or granny develop wrinkles, because the chances are the same thing will happen to you. Have you indulged in the dreaded cigarette, fried your epidermis on Mediterranean beaches, or subjected it to a weather-beaten outdoor life? Hormones affect the skin now as they did in your teenage years, and also if you have ever been pregnant. There are oestrogen receptors in both the epidermis and the dermis. Loss of oestrogen after the menopause contributes to a loss of collagen and hyaluronic acid, and with them the elasticity and moisture-retaining capacities of skin. Collagen may decline as much at 30 per cent in the first five years after the menopause and it keeps dropping thereafter.

Thin, unpadded skin not only sags and wrinkles more easily, it is also more prone to tear and slower to heal. Several studies have demonstrated that HRT, whether pill, patch or topical face cream, delays this process by increasing skin thickness and elasticity and collagen content. People were aware of this as long as 70 years ago, before modern HRT was formulated, and in those days oestrogen and progesterone creams were sold over the counter like cosmetics because of their beneficial effect on the skin. These days pharmacologically active creams are classified as drugs and are on prescription only. Cosmetic products are, by definition, not permitted to contain more than 1 per cent of active ingredients, which means they rarely penetrate more than the outer layer of cells. Nevertheless, moisturizing your skin with some form of cream is better for your skin than leaving it to fend for itself. An American dermatologist called Zoe Dian Draelos (who just happens to market a skin cream that includes 1 per cent of a natural antioxidant called coffee-berry which she claims improves 'skin-fitness'), points out very reasonably that skin health matters at the menopause because anxiety about the skin's appearance can lead to depression, and this may impact negatively on a woman's cardiovascular health. And, while no one would take HRT just to avoid wrinkles (or wouldn't admit to it anyway), nevertheless, I suspect that it is one of the things that makes women taking HRT, despite all they hear about increased health risks, so reluctant to give it up. They are convinced, with some justification, that it is keeping old age at bay.

Hormones and fat

Does the menopause make you fat? Yes, I'm afraid it does – or it can do. Basically it makes it much more difficult to stay slim. All the studies show that the menopause is associated with a progressive increase in weight. But it is more complicated than that. The fat goes on in different places, and it is quite different from youthful or puppy fat. The gain tends to be concentrated round the abdomen, which is the worst place to build up fat from a health point of view. Fat that shows up round the waist also accumulates around the vital organs and is associated with increased cardiovascular risk and diabetes. Flesh becomes softer, less firm – loss of collagen beneath the skin surface again. And the breasts, to quote the singing group Fascinating Aida, 'start their long journey south'.

In youth most women carry their body fat around their hips and thighs, giving them a slightly pear-shaped figure (not all women, I know, but this fat distribution is characteristically female). After the menopause there is a tendency to get more top-heavy: round the middle (made worse when you eventually begin to lose height as you grow older), on your shoulders and on the backs of your arms. Even if you have been successful at controlling your weight when younger, it gets incredibly difficult at this age. 'It's just not fair: I'm eating just the same as I always used to eat, but I'm getting fatter,' you wail.

The way loss of oestrogen affects weight gain is complex. Your metabolism slows gradually as you age. That means that you burn up fewer calories, hence need to eat less, just to stay the same weight. Taking more exercise can help to raise the metabolic rate. And the link to a fall in the production of hormones is demonstrated, once again, in women undergoing an early menopause when their ovaries are removed. They also start to put on weight, even though they are younger than those going through a natural menopause. It appears that oestrogen and another hormone that becomes depleted at the menopause, testosterone, have a knock-on effect on a third hormone, produced in fat cells, called *leptin*. Leptin regulates the relationship between appetite and the rate at which the body burns up energy – the metabolic rate. A loss of oestrogen reduces leptin levels, thereby reducing the calories the body burns, and loss of testosterone – a hormone that plays an important part in men's bodies as well as women's – results in a loss of muscle tissue or lean body mass. Lean body mass burns calories at a higher metabolic rate, so that if you have less of it – as when you spend a long time in bed during illness – you need even fewer calories and you may put on weight while consuming the same amount of food. Exercise boosts muscle bulk and lean body mass and contributes to increasing the metabolic rate.

The leptin connection was neatly demonstrated in a study carried out at Vrije University, Amsterdam. A group of postmenopausal women, all within a normal weight range, were tested for the levels of leptin in their blood, and then half of them were given oestrogen (oestradiol) and the other half a dummy pill – a placebo. After two months the group on the placebo showed no increase in leptin levels but had experienced significant weight gain. The group on HRT, however, had increased their leptin levels by almost 50 per cent and had not gained weight.

HRT does not cause weight gain

You can see why women get so attached to their HRT: improved skin, more comfortable sex, and it's easier to control your weight. A review that looked at the results of 22 different studies found that taking HRT had no effect on women's weight at all. You are over 50, so the gradual slowdown in your metabolism may still make keeping slim more difficult. Added to the fact that the older we get the less inclined we may be to take exercise. Weight control will not be easy, but HRT will make it easier for a while. (And did I mention that it may also prevent hair becoming thinner and changing in texture as a response to depleted oestrogen? What's not to like?)

Hormones and the brain

Women often complain that the menopause is affecting them mentally. They say they are getting forgetful or suffering from 'foggy brain'. Some degree of mental decline is usually considered a natural part of ageing. Short-term memory loss may start to plague you even before you reach 50. (It seems inevitable to me, since the older you get the more there is to remember.) Some 10 per cent of people aged 65 or older have dementia, and this rises to almost 50 per cent of those over 85. The brain undergoes changes as we age. Some parts get smaller and there are signs that the brain processes certain key neurotransmitters less efficiently. Once again there are oestrogen receptors in the brain as there are all over the body, and as in other parts of the body it appears to facilitate blood flow and to be associated with brain activity. (Increased blood flow is what shows up on a magnetic resonance imaging – MRI.) Loss of oestrogen equals loss of blood flow, equals loss of brain activity, equals loss of memory – QED, or so you may think. But not so fast: it turns out not to be demonstrated at all. When you actually subject women who are going through the menopause or after to various tests of mental performance in a research setting, no consistent differences are detected. Nor are there any differences if you test and compare those with and without HRT. In laboratory studies animals given oestrogen consistently perform better on memory tests, but it appears, not for the first time, that human beings are different.

A detailed review of all studies of the effect of HRT on memory and mental function appeared in the *Journal of the American Medical Association* (*JAMA*) in 2001, and no dramatic or consistent trends emerged. In some studies HRT users performed better at verbal recall than non-users, but not in all of them. They showed superior abstract reasoning in some studies, though not in all. In one study they showed better reaction time, in another superior clerical speed. One consistent finding did emerge: those women who showed most improvement on whichever cognitive test while they were on HRT were those women who were experiencing the worst menopausal symptoms when without it. The obvious question arises: were they performing better on HRT simply because they were relieved of all those troublesome symptoms and getting a good night's sleep? Disturbed sleep is known to impair mental performance at any age, and improved sleep has also been shown to improve the disturbed mood, depression and anxiety many women report during the menopause.

A pilot study carried out in the USA after the *JAMA* review as part of Research into Memory, Brain Function and Estrogen Replacement, or REMEMBER, went some way to explaining why various studies turned in conflicting findings for women taking HRT. It related to the age they were when they took it. Do you remember how those women in WHI who took HRT later in life appeared to suffer more damaging effects to their health than those who took it while they were going through the menopause? The same appears to apply with mental performance. The REMEMBER study discovered that those who had taken HRT early tended to outperform those who had never taken it, in verbal fluency, memory and other mental tasks. Whereas those who had taken HRT later in life scored worse than those who had never taken it. *When* you take HRT is crucial for mental as well as physical health. Other studies confirm this effect. Taking HRT at the time of the menopause for as little as three years also lowers the risk of dementia, while taking it long past the menopause puts you at higher risk of mental decline in old age.

There are other complicating factors muddying the waters when it comes to both mood and mental performance at this time. These days, the menopause usually occurs at the crossroads of domestic stress. For mothers with children it coincides with teenagers deserting the nest and going to college. For daughters – and we are all daughters as long as our parents live – the menopause coincides with their parents facing the serious health problems of old age. I once heard a GP say, off the record, 'When I see a woman going through a bad menopause I first check whether her teenage kids are on drugs or granny has become incontinent.'

I hope you are fortunate and are not going through the menopause while being the filling in this generational-stress sandwich. Even if you escape it you may have career or partnership problems to deal with. The fifties can be the cruellest decade. However, if you shoot these rapids there are calm waters beyond.

10

Managing the rest of your life

Looking back on the last four chapters I realize that they make grim reading. In an effort to cover the waterfront on the health risks after the menopause I have given the impression that this change is all for the worse. But it's not. For many women this is a time of turbulence – like shooting the rapids – but it's not like that for everyone, and it doesn't last. You come out onto calm water afterwards.

The goal of this book is to give you an informed perspective on the menopause: a balanced view that represents the relationship between close and distant objects realistically. The butterfly in the foreground appears larger than the tree in the distance; with perspective you see them in proportion. This is how you will view the menopause at 60 or 70. It may dominate your foreground for a few years, but ultimately it will shrink in significance. Think of how you now view your teens: wasn't it awful – the insecurity, the belief that you looked frightful, that the pain of unrequited love would blight your life for ever, that you would never amount to anything at work? Or maybe you can remember how it felt to be a novice mother: the feeling that this new life had taken over yours like a parasite, that you were being engulfed by nappies and half-chewed rusks, and that you would never have an uninterrupted night's sleep again? Even if this was not your experience, or is not your recall, you see what I am getting at. Some periods in your life engulf you while you are going through them, but slip back into the pattern of life's rich tapestry once you have come through to the other side. That is how it will be with the menopause, however ghastly it seems at the time.

Enough philosophy; let's be practical. This is the chapter that concentrates on what you can do to manage your life for the best. Not all these issues will affect you. Some you may already have survived successfully. Others may not concern you, but they will affect some of you some of the time. Skip the bits that don't apply to you.

The perimenopause

One warning sign that the menopause is just round the corner is irregular and heavy periods. If you have heavy periods adopt a resourceful attitude towards sanitary protection. Remember always to have something quick to hand, and don't feel constrained to stick to commercial products. Large quantities of cotton wool can actually be contained in the vagina and come out easily if you have a heavy flow, and will get you through the night or a special occasion. You can also buy an adult version of a baby's protective panties if it makes you feel safer. If a heavy flow is really protracted, or if it happens often, consult your GP. It can be caused by things other than the beginning of the menopause and whatever the cause it can make you anaemic – shortage of the red blood cells that carry oxygen around your body. Your GP can order tests that will confirm the cause and suggest treatment – like putting you on HRT early, which will stabilize the situation, or taking iron capsules to build up your red cells again. There are sources of further information at the end of this book.

Whether your periods become irregular, lighter, less frequent, or just stop, you should continue to use some form of contraception if you are enjoying a regular sex life. A late pregnancy is the last thing most women want to deal with at around 50. Experts recommend that you continue to use contraception for up to two years after your last period. Barrier methods (condom for the man or diaphragm/Dutch cap for the woman) are less successful if vaginal lubrication is in short supply. If you are in the clear for using the contraceptive pill – in other words, you don't smoke, have normal blood pressure, are not overweight and do not have a family history of blood clots or breast cancer – this method has the advantage of providing oestrogen replacement. There is also the 'mini-pill' which is progesterone alone. This method of contraception becomes more effective as women get older.

You should do a thorough personal health check (tabulated) when deciding on how to manage your menopause. It needs to include the health records of the rest of your family because some risks are higher if you have an inherited tendency. (A health checklist that summarizes all those mentioned in these chapters can be found at the back of the book.)

At the menopause: the HRT decision

You can only make informed choices about dealing with the menopause if you have first assessed your personal health. One of the first decisions to make is whether to take HRT or not, because if you are going to do it, you should do it when the menopause first occurs or even before, when it threatens. The HRT decision hinges primarily on the severity of the short-term symptoms that you suffer, and also on whether you are in any of the high-risk groups for adverse long-term health risks. It also depends on your personal priorities and what feels right for you. Take this decision only after you have talked things over thoroughly with your doctor. The voice of authority backs HRT in the short term. The government's Committee on Safety of Medicines says that HRT is helpful for treating symptoms of the menopause, but that women should take the lowest dose that works for them for the shortest amount of time. Helen Buckler, writing in *Endocrinologist* in 2006, is less equivocal: 'No therapy for menopausal vasomotor symptoms has stood the test of time as well as oestrogen therapy. Observational studies continue to show reduced mortality in younger women taking HRT.' She continues, referring to the Women's Health Initiative studies that cast such a pall over HRT in 2002, but which later turned out to be less negative than first appeared:

> In the WHI, the mean age of women recruited was around 63 years, and they were recruited to look at the preventative role of HRT. Most women had no relevant indication to take HRT. The results may not necessarily be relevant to a younger group of postmeno-pausal women and may not apply to different HRT preparations. Although the findings of the study are of major concern, *the HRT preparation used in the study caused neither harm nor benefit to over 99 per cent of the study population.* [The italics are mine.]

I find this last statement tremendously reassuring. As someone who took HRT and felt no untoward outcome, it concerns me that women may not avail themselves of effective therapy for the vaso-motor symptoms of the menopause because of disproportionate fear of very small increases in long-term health risks. This is what another woman, Wilma Prince, from Vossemeer in the Netherlands, writes on the internet:

I have been on HRT for years and tried weaning myself off it several times after reading yet another scare story. However, after a few weeks or sometimes days my life becomes a misery. Hardly any sleep at night, incontinence problems, etc. Fortunately my gynaecologist agrees with me that quality of life is very important. Thanks to HRT, I can lead a normal life, so I am very grateful that it exists.

The *British Medical Journal*'s Best Treatments website adds: 'Some studies show that you're likely to have a greater feeling of wellbeing if you take HRT. You're likely to be less anxious, have more energy, sleep better, and feel more in control and less isolated. You may be able to do more physically and get fewer aches and pains.' In addition to these potential short-term gains, HRT effectively defers many of the longer-term changes that follow the menopause: your vaginal secretions will stick around for a while, you will not have an immediate tendency to put on weight. You will have to deal with them once you come off HRT, but by that time you may have achieved a successful transition to your new postmenopausal life.

By the time you reach this stage of life you have got used to people telling you about the importance of a healthy lifestyle. Hopefully, you won't be reading this book if you have hardened your heart to the message. The menopause is the moment when you can't put things off any longer. Here is a round-up of what you should do to safeguard your health and well-being during the menopause, and ever after.

Some helpful behaviour

1 Stop smoking

There is very little to say about this that smokers have not already heard ad nauseam. It doesn't just make you more likely to get lung cancer – anything from 10 to 20 times more likely – it makes you more likely to get other forms of cancer and also cardiovascular disease and stroke, either of which may kill you as swiftly as lung cancer. At the menopause a woman's risk of getting these conditions goes up. Do something to reduce yours. Give up cigarettes (or cigars, if they are your bag) and every year your health risks will diminish. After a year your risk of heart attack will be half that of a smoker; after ten years your risk of lung cancer will be half that of a smoker; after 15 years your risk of heart attack will be the same as someone who has never smoked. Do it now and plan for a long postmenopause.

2 Take regular exercise

Here again; the message isn't new, but the need to follow it is even greater. There is clear evidence that women who are more active suffer less from the symptoms of the menopause. Not every type of activity leads to an improvement in symptoms. High-impact infrequent exercise can actually make symptoms worse. (It's not all good news for the young either: sports jocks tend to suffer more from injury and from secondary osteoarthritis.) The best exercise in middle to old age (after the menopause) is aerobic, sustained, regular exercise such as swimming or running. The back-stop position is a brisk walk. It can make a really dramatic difference to the quality of your life, although there is a lack of firm evidence as to exactly how much or exactly what sort of exercise you need to take. But if you manage to get the quantity and quality right you can reasonably expect not only improved fitness, but more energy, greater strength and flexibility, less lower back pain and even improved sleep and general well-being – though this is rather difficult to measure. On the health side, you should be at reduced risk of the following age-related conditions.

- Heart attack (risk reduced with as little as 150 calories-worth of physical activity a day: approximately a brisk, one-mile walk)
- Stroke (reduced by 20–40 per cent)
- Type 2 diabetes (reduced by 30 per cent)
- Hip fracture (reduced by 40 per cent)
- Colon cancer (reduced by 10–46 per cent).

And if you haven't been an exerciser so far, your scope for improving your health and quality of life with quite a moderate change in lifestyle is considerable. Research reveals that the unhealthy, unfit elderly can give themselves a real health boost with quite a modest increase in physical activity. You don't need to sweat it out at the gym for hours at a time. Just taking the stairs and walking the dog may be beneficial. National guidelines in the UK and the USA recommend 30 minutes of moderate intensity physical activity at least five (preferably seven) days a week. The definition of moderate intensity that equals 'a brisk walk' is at a rate of about three to four miles an hour. Aim for this level once you hit the menopause if you are not already taking regular, formal exercise. It will do you good, and actually walking, especially in the countryside, or with a dog, is life-enhancing too. And discovering new places to walk is an excellent way to prevent your life contracting.

3 Overhaul your diet

Even if you go on HRT and put off the day when the hormones pack up completely and leave you vulnerable to middle-age spread, now is the time to get into good habits. Check your weight. Body mass index (BMI) is a blunt tool, but it's the best we have. Aim to have a BMI of below 25, and certainly not above 28. Start eating less, but make sure that what you do eat includes foods that do you good, and a minimum of those that do harm. You know the basic principles: lots of fruit and green vegetables; plenty of fish, including oily fish at least twice a week; wholegrain cereals; moderate red meat, and dairy produce; minimal sugar, animal fat and refined starch. Your metabolism is slowing down and your body won't process essential vitamins as well as when you were younger. Pay particular attention to three things.

Calcium

Calcium is especially important if you are in a high-risk group for developing brittle bones. At the menopause your daily requirement of calcium needs to double to 1,200 or even 1,500 mg a day. The obvious source of calcium is dairy produce, but since you will also be trying to limit the amount of saturated (animal) fats in your diet so that you don't add to your risk of developing cardiovascular disease and cancer, you should keep full-cream milk, yoghurt and cheese to a minimum. Two glasses (400 ml) of semi-skimmed milk, two 150-gram pots of low-fat yogurt plus 30 grams of cheese should supply an average daily calcium requirement. And if you don't particularly like dairy produce there is also a lot of calcium in sardines (you eat the bones), sesame seeds and dried figs, among other things.

Essential vitamins

It becomes more difficult for the body to absorb vitamins after the menopause. Some vitamins help combat the short-term symptoms of the menopause, others combat long-term health risks like cardiovascular disease and osteoporosis. Vitamin B2, found in liver, kidney, mushrooms and soya beans, has been shown to relieve perimenopausal headaches. Soya is one of the plant oestrogens (phytoestrogens) we discussed earlier, which acts in a similar way to natural oestradiol or HRT. Some studies suggest that adding soya to the diet can reduce hot flushes by as much as 40 per cent. (One theory is that a soya-rich diet could explain why Japanese women going through the menopause suffer less from hot flushes than western women.) Vitamin E is another alternative to HRT that is reported to relieve hot flushes, and to be protective against heart attacks, Alzheimer's disease, and cancer. It is found in vegetable oils, nuts and seeds. Vitamin B6 and vitamin B12 (folic acid) can be found in leafy green vegetables, liver, eggs and fish, and lower the risk of heart disease, blood clots and osteoporosis, and may even alleviate depression. Vitamin D is also absolutely vital if your body is to absorb calcium efficiently. Achieving adequate vitamin D through diet alone is pretty difficult. The best source is sunlight, often in short supply in Great Britain and particularly in Scotland. You need at least 20 minutes of high-angle sunlight (late March to September) over a generous area of bare skin to maintain adequate vitamin D levels. Sunbathe judiciously (avoiding burning) when this is possible, and take a supplement when it is not. In your fifties you probably need at least 500 IU (international units) a day, rising to 1,000 IU a day according to some experts, or even more, by the time you reach 70. Summing up: you can see that vegetables, liver, fish, low-fat dairy produce, nuts and seeds are all good for you at the menopause and that if you are in any doubt it does no harm to take a multivitamin pill, or at very least a vitamin D supplement.

Alcohol

Alcohol becomes more difficult for the body to process after the menopause. Women need to watch the sauce at all ages; the female liver is not as good at clearing the toxins in alcohol as the male. After the menopause the liver becomes less efficient, and in addition, you will probably be eating less, so watching your units becomes even more important. What's more, alcohol, cola, strong coffee or tea and spicy food can all aggravate hot flushes. You don't need to become a killjoy, but binge-drinking is a killer. People who manage to drink moderately (three units a day or less for women) usually lead healthier lives. Join the club.

4 Nurture your sex life

If you put 'sex and the menopause' into Google it offers you more than three million hits. Most sites urge you not to think that sex stops at the menopause. To find practical advice on how to make sure this doesn't happen, you have to dig deeper. You have already learned that maintaining sexual activity acts to preserve the lining and muscles of your vagina. You are not obliged to engage in sexual athletics that involve hanging from the chandelier; the kind of sexual activity you engage in is a matter of individual choice. At 50 you have nothing to prove, and nothing to lose. Hopefully you have learned what you enjoy and what you can leave to the realms of the imagination. (If you are trying sex with a new partner novel excitements could put in an appearance.) But either way, if you have enjoyed a healthy sex life so far there is certainly no reason to give up just because your hormones are on the wane and you can no longer get pregnant.

It's true that some women have a problem with discomfort in intercourse and a shortage of natural lubrication. Any nice-smelling cream can be substituted, and there are some designed specifically for the purpose available from specialist outlets. There is, after all, more to sexual pleasure than intercourse, and after the menopause the *clitoris* – that delightful little female appendage so easily accessible to hands and other forms of stimulation – is still available for duty. In fact the majority (at least 70 per cent) of women, according to studies, do not reach orgasm through vaginal intercourse or vagina-only stimulation anyway. Which is not surprising since, compared with the clitoris and the area surrounding the opening of the vagina – more properly called the *vulva* – the internal walls of the vagina are not rich in nerve endings. Stephanie Taylor, founder of the company Passion8, sells and vouches for the effectiveness of several creams. Eden Bliss is a silicone lubricant that can be used to relieve dryness and make intercourse friction-free. Replens, a bioadhesive moisturizer, claims to rehydrate the tissues, and one called informatively 'Oh my clitoral stimulating cream' improves peripheral circulation when rubbed into the area around the clitoris.

The most important erogenous zone remains the brain. This is where all sexual excitement is generated or processed. There are books written expressly to turn women on, and it occurs to me that erotic fantasies are probably one area where books will never be overtaken by the internet. If you are part of a stable partnership you may both have to be more patient and more inventive to keep the spark alive. Websites to stimulate the sexual imagination are listed at the back of the book.

If you are single, cultivate an open mind not only about what you do but whom you do it with. There is nothing wrong with starting a relationship with a younger man just as, for centuries, older men have got involved with younger women. (Let's face it, the older you get the more younger people there are about.) At the time I am writing this the singer Madonna, at 50, has found herself a dishy young lover 22 years younger than she is. Provided you are secure in yourself, there is clearly no reason why it shouldn't be a success: he has youth and vigour; you have knowhow and experience, and fewer hang-ups than a 20-year-old.

5 Enlarge your horizons

This advice applies more to the years following the menopause than to the event itself. Many women, especially career women, are in their prime in their early fifties. Hopefully their horizons will continue to expand professionally for at least ten years, maybe even into retirement and beyond. But it can be a problem for housewives, or those whose lives have been centred on children and the family. The time when the children leave home and start having lives, homes and families of their own can be particularly hard. And it comes at about the same time as the menopause. The 'empty-nest syndrome' is something that every mother faces to some extent. If it coincides with having to become a carer for the older generation – your own parents – it is particularly difficult. There is the danger that your whole life becomes overwhelmed by looking after other people. Don't let it. Even a good mother and a good daughter deserves time for herself.

Horizons are an important part of perspective. Keeping them broad and open means keeping up with friends and having activities outside the home, which takes more effort as you get older. Beware the temptation to say 'It's too far' or 'It's too late'. It's never too far or too late to keep an old friend or make a new one. It's important too to make friends who are younger than you. Nothing is more depressing than reaching your sixties and starting to go to more funerals than weddings and christenings. It's one of the few advantages of being a single parent (or becoming one, if you don't start out as one). You are less confined to contemporary friendships. You make friends of your children and your children's friends, and all the age groups in between. Younger friends, like younger lovers, keep *you* young. And they are around longer when you get old too.

The same goes for interests and activities. Take up new ones; hold on to old ones. No problem if you enjoy the things of the mind: books, music, theatre and film. Things you can both watch or join in. The danger here is in the box in the corner. Watching TV is the number one activity for both sexes in this country. There is some great stuff on UK television and it makes interesting material to discuss with friends afterwards, but it can become a rather addictive drug. Try to get out of the house and see a film, listen to music, join a book club, watch sport or take up golf, if you can afford it. If you are already someone who enjoys outdoor activities you should find this easy. You may have to scale down a bit. If you played squash or tennis in your thirties, golf may suit you better after the menopause. If you used to run the marathon plenty of evidence shows that you may still be able to do it, but it will be adequate for you to take regular brisk walks if you don't want to indulge in all that sweating any more. The top activity among women in the UK is walking, followed by swimming and keep fit or dance classes. A dance class has the great advantage that you can do it with a friend or partner.

One outdoor activity increasing in popularity these days is gardening, particularly growing fruit and vegetables. More people without gardens are applying for allotments, which until recently had been in decline. There is something extremely satisfying about eating things you have grown yourself. You can do it alone or with a partner, and if you are alone, you soon make friends at the allotments. It's not difficult, it doesn't have to take up a lot of space, and there is loads of helpful information around about how to get started. (There are useful contacts at the back of this book.) Adventurous souls have been known to take up bee-keeping, or even chickens, though this could be a responsibility too far if you have just emptied your nest of children and fancy the idea of doing more travelling. Looking after plants and animals seems to chime with something nurturing in women. At least, I have never found the woman who got an equal satisfaction out of killing things – pheasants, foxes or fish. Follow Voltaire's excellent advice and 'cultivate your garden' for a contented postmenopause.

Epilogue

I have introduced a few women going through the menopause in the course of this book. I thought you might like to know how things went with some of them.

My friend Maria – the one who went through it hardly noticing it was happening, and without taking a thing to treat it – has had a few problems. Now entering her seventies, she has, like her mother, got delicate bones and has developed osteoporosis. She is taking alendronic acid and has so far avoided anything more troublesome than a hairline fracture of the ankle that required MRI to reveal itself. She has also had breast cancer. But they caught it early. She sailed through surgery and radiotherapy with her customary buoyancy, and has been free of it now for five years. She still works, and still enjoys sex, if it comes her way. She has a rich life, full of friends and activities.

Jane – who had such heavy periods at the perimenopause that her doctor prescribed iron pills to correct her anaemia, and put her on HRT to stabilize the bleeding – stayed on HRT for 20 years, and her GP didn't take her off it until, at nearly 70, her blood pressure started to rise. She had reduced her dose to half-pills taken every other day. When she stopped the hot flushes returned, but they were manageable. Her health is good – the BP is now controlled with drugs – and she is still working in the competitive profession of public relations. She married for the second time at 70 so I rather suppose the sex is OK too.

Joanna – who had suffered badly from premenstrual tension and painful intercourse at the menopause – was advised against HRT because she was a smoker (she has cut back, but still has the occasional guilty drag) and also because her mother had had breast cancer. She had bad hot flushes and tried one alternative therapy after another without any success. Finally her doctor prescribed SSRIs which helped a little. Then, after three or four bad years, medically and domestically, she surprised us all by leaving her husband and moving in with another woman. Her life was transformed. She started a new business with the partner, and they go on adventure holidays snorkelling or on camels in the Sahara. So far, cross fingers, no breast cancer, though she has annual mammograms.

My mother lived to be nearly 90. She was one of those people who confound the statistics: took no medication and had excellent health, yet still enjoyed the occasional Scotch and a cigarette until the end. When my father died in his sixties she started visiting opera houses all over Europe. She lived in her own house, with a large garden, and continued to teach the piano until two months before the end. She was out in the garden pruning the raspberries during her very last summer. My most abiding memory of her is coming in from the garden in her old gardening gloves with a leaf in her auburn hair.

There is a lot of life to enjoy yet after the menopause.

Glossary

Anaemia/anaemic A reduction in the number of red blood cells, reducing the blood's ability to carry oxygen and other nutrients around the body.

Angina Chest pain caused by reduced flow of blood to the heart muscle.

Atheroma Abnormal fatty deposits that accumulate within the walls of arteries.

Atherosclerosis Clogging or hardening of arteries or blood vessels caused by atheroma.

Arteriosclerosis Hardening, narrowing or loss of elasticity in large or medium-sized arteries or blood vessels.

Atrial fibrillation An irregular heart rhythm in the upper chambers of the heart; a risk factor for stroke.

Autoimmune system The mechanism by which the body recognizes 'self' from 'foreign'. In autoimmune conditions like rheumatoid arthritis or diabetes this system reacts against its own tissues or cells as though they were foreign, and damages them.

Bisphosphonates A class of drugs, including alendronic acid, that slow bone resorption; used to treat brittle bones.

Cardiovascular disease Disorders of the heart and circulation.

Carotid arteries The major arteries in the neck supplying blood to the brain.

Cervix, cervical The neck of the womb that projects into the back of the vagina. Changes in the cells lining the opening may signal increased risk of cervical cancer.

Clitoris A small, erect organ in front of the opening of the vagina sensitive to sexual excitement.

Colorectal cancer Cancer that affects the colon (lower bowel) or rectum.

Comparator A treatment used in a clinical trial as the base-line against which a new drug or treatment's effectiveness is measured. It may be either the current treatment or a dummy, or sugar pill – a placebo.

Corticosteroids Potent, anti-inflammatory hormones produced naturally in the body or synthetically for use as drugs.

Coronary arteries The blood vessels communicating directly with the heart that provide it with oxygen-rich blood.

C-reactive protein (CPR) A by-product and indicator of inflammation, detectable in a blood test.

Cyst A small, usually harmless sealed sac that forms in the body, usually filled with fluid. Cysts sometimes disappear spontaneously, but at other times may be removed surgically.

Cystitis Inflammation of the tract leading to the bladder.

Defecation The elimination of (usually solid) waste through the anus.

Diabetes An autoimmune condition where the body is unable to produce or handle the human hormone insulin, and is thereby unable to absorb carbohydrates from the diet. In type 1 diabetes no natural insulin is produced and must be supplied by regular injections. In type 2 the body becomes unable to handle naturally produced insulin, but it may be treatable with oral drugs. This type is associated with obesity and adds to the risk of heart attack and stroke.

Drospirenone A progesterone-like manufactured hormone used in contraceptives and recently in HRT.

Dual-energy X-ray absorbtiometry (DEXA) The gold standard for measuring bone density using low-energy X-ray.

Dysmenorrhoea Pain during the monthly period.

Embolism A loose clot, or air bubble or other particle that blocks a blood vessel.

Embryo An organism in the early stage of its development prior to birth. In humans it covers from when a sperm fertilizes an egg until the eighth week of pregnancy when it becomes a foetus (US fetus), see below.

Endometrium The mucous membrane lining the womb.

Endometriosis The growth of the tissue that lines the womb in other parts of the body such as the ovaries, which causes pain during menstruation.

Epidermis The outer layer of skin.

Equine Derived from, or relating to, horses.

Fallopian tubes Two finger-like tubes, also known as oviducts, which connect the ovaries with the womb. The sperm and egg meet in the Fallopian tubes (named after the sixteenth-century anatomist who identified them) and carry fertilized eggs to the womb.

Foetus The word for the unborn baby from the eighth week of pregnancy until birth.

Follicle A small sac-like group of cells. The ovarian follicle is the sac in which an egg (ovum) develops prior to fertilization.

Follicle-stimulating hormone (FSH) A hormone produced in the pituitary gland that controls oestrogen production by the ovaries.

Hormone replacement therapy (HRT) A pharmaceutically produced combination of oestrogens and progestogens that treats the symptoms of the menopause.

Hormones Naturally produced chemicals that affect cells in other parts of the body.

Homocysteine A factor found in the blood which if high is thought to be a risk factor for blood clots, heart attack and stroke.

Hyaluronic acid A naturally occurring gel-like substance in skin that retains moisture.

Hyperlipidaemia Abnormally high levels of fats in the bloodsteam.

Hypertension High blood pressure (BP): symptomless, but if above 140/90 a risk factor for kidney disease, heart disease and stroke.

Hypoglycaemia Low levels of sugar in the bloodstream; usually as a result of not eating.

Hysterectomy The surgical removal of the womb.

In vitro fertilization (IVF) Combining sperm and egg in the laboratory prior to re-implantion in the womb.

Leptin A hormone that plays a key role in regulating energy intake and energy expenditure.

Luteinizing hormone (LH) A hormone produced by the pituitary gland that stimulates the release of oestrogen from the ovaries, causing ovulation.

Magnetic resonance imaging (MRI) An imaging technique that uses magnetic fields to take cross-sectional pictures of structures in the body or brain.

Mammogram Diagnostic imaging of the breast by X-ray or ultrasound.

Metabolic syndrome A combination of risk factors that increase the risk of developing cardiovascular disease and diabetes.

Menarche The time of the first menstrual period.

Mucous membrane/mucosa The lining of body cavities like the mouth, nose, vagina and the digestive tract.

Neurotransmitter Chemicals that transmit impulses between nerve cells.

Noradrenaline A stress hormone associated with arousal and the fight-or-flight response; raises heart rate, triggering a release of glucose and increased blood flow to skeletal muscles.

Occlusion, occluded Blockage, blocked.

Oestradiol The most potent form of natural oestrogen, produced in the ovaries until the menopause and synthesized in the laboratory for use as hormone replacement.

Oestrogens, unopposed oestrogen Form of oestrogen produced in a laboratory; used alone to treat menopausal symptoms in women who have had a hysterectomy.

Oophorectomy (bilateral oophorectomy) The surgical removal of both ovaries.

Osteoblasts Cells that create new bone.

Osteoclasts Cells that absorb bone.

Osteoporosis Loss of bone density resulting in brittle, easily broken bones.

Ovulation The release of an egg from the ovaries into the Fallopian tubes.

Ovum (plural, ova) The early development stage of the female egg before it has been fertilized, also called a gamete.

Perimenopause The period just before the natural menopause when oestrogen production is reduced.

Pessary A vaginal suppository; gelatinous formulation of medication that dissolves once lodged in the vagina. (The term is also used for a contraceptive diaphragm or for a device that supports the neck of a prolapsed womb.)

Pituitary gland A pea-sized gland at the base of the brain that secretes follicle-stimulating hormone (FSH) and luteinizing hormone (LH) and thereby controls the menstrual cycle.

Placebo A dummy or sugar pill given to one group in a clinical trial to conceal which patients are receiving the active drug and which are not.

Premenstrual tension (PMT) Also known as premenstrual syndrome; a collection of physical and psychological symptoms experienced by some women just before their monthly period.

Progesterone A hormone secreted by the ovaries that prepares the womb to receive a fertilized egg.

Progestogens Laboratory-manufactured versions of progesterone used in HRT.

Prostate gland A gland that encircles the male urethra and produces some of the fluid in semen.

Quiescent Of the endometrial lining (or volcanoes), in a state of tranquil repose; dormant.

Selective oestrogen receptor modulator (SERMs) A class of drugs that blocks oestrogen receptors in some but not other parts of the body.

Selective serotonin reuptake inhibitors (SSRIs) A class of anti-depressant drugs that blocks the reabsorption of the neurotransmitter serotonin in the brain, thereby increasing its beneficial affect on mood.

Subcutis The deepest layer of skin, which contains mostly fat cells and acts as padding, insulation and an energy store.

Testosterone A potent hormone responsible for masculine traits, produced in the testes in men, but in lesser quantities by the ovaries in women.

Thrombosis (thrombus) A clot in a blood vessel that, if it breaks loose, may cause a heart attack or stroke.

Thromboembolism A thrombus that causes a blockage of a major blood vessel. If it blocks the pulmonary artery it is a pulmonary embolism.

Thyroid A gland responsible for temperature regulation and other metabolic functions.

Tubal ligation A form of female sterilization achieved by closing the Fallopian tubes so that an ovum cannot reach the womb.

Ultrasound The use of sound waves bounced off different body tissues to build up a picture, sometimes a moving picture; also called sonography.

Urethra The duct through which urine is expelled from the bladder. (In the male it is also a conduit for semen.)

Vasomotor (symptoms) Increases in the diameter of subcutaneous blood vessels, causing, among other things, a sudden flush and sweat.

Vulva A collective term for the external female genitalia; includes the clitoris, labia and the opening of the vagina.

Appendix

Draw up your risk profile

Health is an individual thing; none of us is exactly the same as another. But we have a number of things in common and a number of differences that research has shown contribute to health changes and health risks after the menopause.

You can take this check list seriously and tick the risks that apply to you and see how you score – like a 'Now check your rating' quiz in a magazine – or you can simply look through it totting up in your mind where you are at risk and where you appear to be in the clear. This choice is probably less likely to make you anxious. Some of these risk factors can be modified by changing your behaviour. Read those even if you pass over the risks connected with your inherited constitution and what has happened to you in the past. We have marked risk factors you, or your doctor by prescribing, can correct with an asterisk like this *.

Risk factors for having a heart attack

- Bad lipid/cholesterol profile*
- High blood pressure*
- Smoking*
- Diabetes*
- Obesity*
- Level of C-reactive protein in blood
- Level of homocysteine in blood
- High stress levels*.

Risk factors for having a stroke

- High blood pressure*
- Smoking*
- Diabetes*
- Narrowing of carotid (brain) blood vessels
- Atrial fibrillation
- Obesity*.

Factors that increase the risk of breast cancer (in order of significance)

- Menopause occurred after you were 55 (doubles your risk from average)
- No children before the age of 30
- Obesity following the menopause*
- Periods started before the age of 11
- Drink more than three units of alcohol each day*
- Combined HRT for more than five years*
- A mother *or* sister is diagnosed with breast cancer before the age of 40
- A mother *or* sister and a more distant relative but from the same side of the family are diagnosed with it after the age of 50
- Two close (mother/sister) relatives are diagnosed after the age of 50
- Two close (mother/sister) relatives diagnosed before average age of 50
- One close, plus one more distant relative, average age 50, diagnosed
- Three or more relatives of any kind or diagnosed at any age.

Risk factors for osteoporosis

- Early menopause
- A female relative already has osteoporosis
- You are exceptionally thin or tall
- Diet deficient in calcium and vitamin D*
- Skin rarely exposed to sunshine*
- Smoking*
- Not taking regular exercise*
- Drinking a lot of strong coffee*
- Drinking more than 3 units of alcohol a day*
- Taking corticosteroid drugs (anti-inflammatory)
- Low bone density.

Further reading

MacGregor, Anne (2006). *Understanding Menopause and HRT*. London: Family Doctor Publications.

Murray, Jenni (2003). *Is it Me or is it Hot in Here? A Modern Woman's Guide to the Menopause*. London: Vermilion.

*Parker-Pope, Tara (2006). *HRT: Everything You Need to Know to Untangle the Controversy, Understand Your Options, Make Your Own Choices*. Kutztown, PA: Rodale.

Petras, Kath (2000). *The Premature Menopause Book*. New York: Avon Books.

*Rees, Margaret; Purdie, David; Hope, Sally (eds) (2006). *The Menopause: What You Need to Know*. Marlow: British Menopause Society.

*Uebelacker, Carol (2004). *Exploring Your Options: Making Informed Decisions About Hormones: Practical Answers for Women in Pre-, Peri- and Post Menopause*. Bloomington, IN: iUniverse.

*author recommendation

Useful addresses and websites

Menopause organizations

British Menopause Society
4–6 Eton Place
Marlow
Bucks SL7 2QA
Tel.: 01628 890199
Website: www.thebms.org.uk

Menopause Amarant Trust
80 Lambeth Road
London SE1 1PW
Advice Line: 09068 660620
British Medical Journal's 'Best Treatments' website
http://besthealth.bmj.com/btuk/home.jsp

Premature menopause

Daisy Network
Website: www.daisynetwork.org.uk
The Daisy Network Premature Menopause Support Group is a registered charity run by volunteers and members to help those women who are experiencing the menopause before they are 45.

International Premature Ovarian Failure Association
Website: www.pofsupport.org

A North American organization with its headquarters in Alexandria, Virginia, with support groups across the country: newsletters and other publications are available.

www.womenshealthsolutions.co.uk

A site run by Ethicon, a division of Johnson & Johnson, to give help and information on a range of health problems affecting women. A careline is provided: 0800 783 9162.

Cancer

Cancer Research UK
PO Box 123
Lincoln's Inn Fields
London WC2A 3PX
Tel.: 020 7121 6699 (supporter services)
020 7242 0200 (switchboard)
Website: www.cancerresearch.org.uk

From the website given, other websites can be accessed; one includes a 'chat' facility. For breast cancer risks, try <www.cancerhelp.org.uk>

Sexual problems and pleasures

Office for Gender and Health, University of Melbourne
This office has undertaken the Melbourne Women's Midlife Health Project, which is a study of women's health during midlife and the menopause.
Website: www.psychiatry.unimelb.edu.au/midlife

General

Website: www.allotment.org.uk
This website provides an index of allotments available and much other information.

Website: www.patientuk.co.uk
This is a good, all-purpose health website: its statement that it supplies 'the same health information as provided by GPs to patients during consultation' says it all, except, of course, it is not specifically geared to you as an individual.

Index

alcohol 72, 76, 92–3
alendronic acid 74, 76
alternative and complementary
  remedies 2
Alzheimer's disease 92
Amarant Trust xi
anaemia 3, 11
anxiety attacks 27
Aristotle 11, 20
arteriosclerosis 35
atherosclerosis 50
autoimmune system 23

bisphosphonates 74
blood clots 55
  development of 54
  thrombosis 50
blood lipids
  hormones and 51–2
  hyperlipidemia 50
blood pressure
  hypertension 50
  importance of 52–4
bones
  see osteoporosis
breast cancer 75
  effect of Tamoxifen 22
  HRT and 64–5
  risk factors 61–4
  screening for 24–5, 60–1, 64
breasts, tenderness of 27
British Menopause Society xi, 58
Brown-Séquard, Charles-Edouard
  16–17
Buckler, Helen 88

calcium 71–2, 74, 76, 91
  Vitamin D 92
cancer
  biopsies 26
  breast 24–5, 43, 46, 49, 59, 61–4,
    75
  cervical 24
  colon 45, 59, 66, 90

diet and 92
family history of 47
HRT and 43, 64–7
incidence of 59
oestrogen and 6
ovaries 67
restoring fertility after 22
screening for 59, 60–1, 64
smoking and 89–90
cervical smears 24
cold hands and feet 27
Committee on Safety of Medicines 88
concentration and memory 27
contraceptive pills 87
contraceptives
  cancer and 62, 64, 66, 67
cystitis 27

Daisy Network 24
depression 1
diet and nutrition 76
  osteoporosis 72
  weight control 82–3
digestive system
  menopausal symptoms 27
Draelos, Zoe Dian 81
drugs
  bone loss and 73–5
  SSRIs 35
  standards for studies 41–3
  see also herbal remedies; hormone
    replacement therapy (HRT)

endometriosis 23
endometrium 5
  cancer of 7, 41, 66–7, 75
environmental pollution 23
exercise 76, 90–1

fatigue 9
fats
  leptin levels 82–3
fertility and childbearing
  after cancer treatment 22

dangers of 12–13
as illness 16
in vitro fertilization 24
fibroids 25
Forever Feminine (Wilson) 17–18

Galen 11
genetic factors
age at menopause 20

headache 9
Healy, David
The Antidepressant Era 43
heart and cardiovascular system 29
diet and 92
exercise and 90
HRT and 41, 43–4, 56–8
menopause and heart attacks 49
palpitations 9, 27
risk factors 55–6
terminology of 50
herbal remedies
phytoestrogens 36
Hill, Austin Bradford 42–3
hormone replacement therapy (HRT)
attitudes towards x, 29–30
blood clots and 54
blood lipids and 51–2
blood pressure and 54
cancers and 25, 64–5, 64–7
composition of 31
deciding on 2
development of Premarin 17–18
forms of 32–4
hot flushes and 8
long-term effect x–xi
making your choice 88–9
Nurses' Health Study 41
opposition to 18
osteoporosis and 73–4
risks and benefits of 39–46
skin and 79–82
timing of 56–7
treating menopause 30
your own health profile 46–8
hormones
blood lipids and 51–2
blood tests for 25
brain processes and 84–5

effect of 4
follicle-stimulating hormone (FSH)
6, 7
heart disease and 49
identification of 16–17
luteinizing hormone (LH) 6
noradrenaline 8
progesterone 6–7, 19, 31
progestogen 19, 30, 31, 34, 66–7
skin and 79–82
testosterone 31, 37, 82–3
vaginal dryness 37
see also oestrogen
hot flushes 1, 27, 57
body thermostat and 7–8
drinks and 93
HRT and x
treatments for 35
HRT: Everything you need to know
(Parker Pope) 30
hypoglycaemia 27

joint pain 27
*Journal of the American Medical
Association* (JAMA) 84–5

Leake, John 12

Melbourne, University of 77, 78–9
men and andropause 11
menopause
age variations 20–1
attitudes towards 15–16
drug treatments 30–6
early 21–4, 82
family and career contexts 85
historical views of 11–12, 16
as illness 18
in life's context ix–xii, 94–6
looking back on 86
medical tests and 24–6
as natural 28–30
other animals and 13–14
the perimenopause 9
postmenopausal women ix, 12,
13–15
symptoms of 1–4, 27–8, 36–8
theories of 12–14
menstrual periods

changes in 87
continued with HRT 2
end of 1–2, 3
hormones and 4–7
irregularity of 27
loss of blood 3
mental ability and concentration 84–5
Million Women study xi, 67
mood changes 1, 4, 27

National Institute for Health and Clinical Excellence (NICE) 63–4
Nurses' Health Study 41, 57
nutrition and diet 20, 91–2
age at menopause 20

oestrogen
bones and 69–70
endometrial cancer 66–7
heart disease and 49
hot flushes 7–8
in HRT 31, 32–4
medical development of 17–18, 40–1
phytoestrogens 36, 92
role in reproduction 4–7
sexual activity and 77–8
Tamoxifen and 22
vaginal dryness and 9
osteoporosis x, 29, 97
ageing process 68–9
bone density scans 26
diet and 91–2
exercise and fractures 90
HRT and 2, 44–5
oestrogens and 69–70
risk factors 71–3
symptoms of 70–1
treatment for 73–6
ovaries
autoimmune system and 23
cancer of 67
cysts 22, 25
egg production 30
oestrogen and 6
premature ovarian failure 21–4
release of eggs 68

removal of 21–2

Packer, Craig 13–14
Parker Pope, Tara 57
HRT: Everything you need to know 30, 46
on osteoporosis 70
Parkhill, Tom xi
phytoestrogens 36
Premarin
see hormone replacement therapy (HRT)
premenstrual tension 3
Prince, Wilma 88–9

randomized controlled trial (RCT) 41
reproduction
ovulation 6–7
role of hormones 4–7

selective oestrogen receptor modulators (SERM) 75
selective serotonin reuptake inhibitors (SSRIs) 35–6
sexual activity 77–9
libido and 37
menopausal symptoms 9
nurturing 93–4
painful 36–7
symptoms of menopause 4
vaginal dryness 4, 9, 27, 36–7, 57, 77–8
skin
anatomy of 80
hormones and 79–82
thinning of 3
sleep disturbance 9, 27, 57, 85
smoking 89–90
age at menopause 20
osteoporosis and 72
stress incontinence 37–8
strokes 90
HRT and 43–4
strontium ranelate 75
Study of Women's Health Across the Nation (SWAN) 15

Taylor, Stephanie 93–4

thyroid tests 25
tuberculosis drug study 42–3

Voronoff, Serge 17
Vrije University 83

Wake Forest University Nurses Study
  xi
Wayne State University 8
weight gain 9

Wilbrush, Joel 12
Wilson, Robert
  Forever Feminine 17–18
womb
  exam of lining 25
  hysteroscopy 26
Women's Health Initiative (WHI) xi,
  56–7, 88
    HRT study 43–6
    osteoporosis 74